Praise for *Lasting Wellbeing*

"This book is a powerful companion for anyone seeking deeper joy, gratitude, and inner peace. Bloom beautifully blends science-backed practices with accessible guidance, inviting readers into a more aligned way of living."

—Alexandra Elle, *New York Times* bestselling author of *How We Heal*

"Guided by science and packed with practical exercises, this phenomenal book teaches anyone how to achieve wellbeing. It is vital reading for experiencing greater joy and meaning in life."

—Scott Sonenshein, *New York Times* bestselling coauthor of *Joy at Work* and author of *Stretch*

"Engaging and easy to read, this book offers a tool kit of science-based practices for boosting and sustaining wellbeing. Matt Bloom offers actionable insights that readers can put to use right away."

—Daniel Cable, author of *Exceptional* and *Alive at Work*

Also by Matt Bloom

Flourishing in Ministry

Lasting Wellbeing

SCIENCE-BASED PRACTICES FOR TRANQUILITY, AUTHENTICITY, MEANING, AND JOY

Matt Bloom, PhD

BENBELLA

BenBella Books, Inc.
Dallas, TX

This book is for informational purposes only. It is not intended to serve as a substitute for professional medical advice. The author and publisher specifically disclaim any and all liability arising directly or indirectly from the use of any information contained in this book. A healthcare professional should be consulted regarding your specific medical situation. Any product mentioned in this book does not imply endorsement of that product by the author or publisher.

BENBELLA

BenBella Books, Inc.
8080 N. Central Expressway
Suite 1700
Dallas, TX 75206
benbellabooks.com
Send feedback to feedback@benbellabooks.com

BenBella is a federally registered trademark.

Printed in the United States of America
10 9 8 7 6 5 4 3 2 1

Library of Congress Control Number: 2026002025
ISBN 9781637748787 (hardcover)
ISBN 9781637748794 (electronic)

Editing by Leah Wilson and Clara Tamez
Copyediting by James Fraleigh
Proofreading by Karen Wise and Mary White
Indexing by WordCo. Indexing Services
Text design and composition by PerfecType, Nashville, TN
Cover design by Sarah Avinger
Cover image © Adobe Stock / beerlogoff
Printed by Lake Book Manufacturing

To all of the wonderful people who participated in my research.

And most of all, to Kim.

Contents

Contents

A Note About Quotes and Citations

The people whose quotes and life histories appear in this book were part of my research. To protect their privacy, I have used pseudonyms and changed identifying details. The quotes are drawn directly from interview transcripts, field notes, and conversations my team and I had as part of our research. The quotes adhere closely to what was said, but they are often not exact. When spoken words are written verbatim, verbal gestures and conversational fillers used in ordinary talk are included, which can make people sound weird or disjointed on the page. I have removed these extraneous words but have always retained the sense and meaning of what each speaker said.

CHAPTER ONE

Starting Well

A few years ago, I was having trouble with my left shoulder, a condition called adhesive capsulitis that is commonly known as frozen shoulder. After ignoring it for several months, I did what perhaps you would have done: I searched the internet for remedies. The results were bewildering. There were various stretching routines, of course, and several different kinds of yoga, but also Rolfing, Reiki, Feldenkrais therapy, trigger point therapy, Gurdjieff movements, a protocol called PAILs and RAILs, therapeutic massage, bee sting therapy (yes, really!), and quite a few others. I had no idea how to select the right approach, so I opted for traditional physical therapy.

After eight expensive months with little improvement, I stopped. Unsure what to do next, I resigned myself to having a permanently frozen shoulder. Until, that is, I stumbled upon a medical book offering one of the remedies in the list above. I followed its instructions, and within a couple of months my shoulder was unfrozen. It remains that way today.

I am not identifying it because I don't know why it worked or even if it worked; maybe my relief came through a placebo effect. Maybe my shoulder healed on its own and the "remedy" did nothing. Or maybe I just lucked out, because following the book's instructions could have made things worse. What I needed in my pain and bewilderment was a guide to help me navigate all the possible options so I could focus on those with solid scientific support. From there, I could find approaches that suited me best in terms of fitting my lifestyle and personal preferences. For example, although research shows that massages are a good remedy, I don't like them, so I looked for something else.

You may face similar confusion when you try to find ways of sustaining your emotional, mental, and spiritual health, which together make up your wellbeing. Effective guidance is hard to come by. A recent survey showed that four out of five American adults were looking for ways to boost their wellbeing, but almost half felt lost in their search.[1] Another poll found that nearly 90 percent of young adults reported experiencing high stress but didn't know how to alleviate it.[2]

One cause of this confusion is that wellbeing has become a multibillion-dollar industry, so there is a torrent of information to slog through. This endeavor is perilous because the deluge is a mix of some very good information, some worthless ideas, and some insidiously harmful advice. Furthermore, the pervasive and aggressive marketing of wellbeing "remedies" propagates fictions like "With the right wellbeing practices, lifelong happiness is attainable," "Hack your brain and unlock your limitless potential," and "All you need to flourish is inside you." None of those claims are true and any can be hazardous. It's extremely difficult for most people to distinguish the helpful guidance from the useless and dangerous.

To navigate this chaos, you need a trustworthy, knowledgeable guide, one that can help you make the right decisions for yourself and the people you care about. Science provides that guide. Research insights can help you truly understand your wellbeing and empower you to find self-care practices that will fit your lifestyle and preferences.

This book, which is based upon my nearly thirty years of research on wellbeing, will help you understand and use what that science has to offer. As a professor at the University of Notre Dame, I have been part of a global community of wellbeing scholars, and you will find the research of many of these people in this book along with my own.

To research this subject, I traveled around the United States and to more than twenty-five other countries to study the wellbeing of people who worked in the helping and healing professions, including international humanitarian workers, physicians and healthcare professionals, clergy, and public-school teachers. Wellbeing researchers often study those in "extreme" conditions because learning how people in these difficult and demanding situations adjust, cope, and thrive provides important insights for those of us whose living and working conditions are more "normal." Just as studying how elite athletes train provides the groundwork for the kinds of exercise practices we can use, my research into the wellbeing of these people provided similarly important foundations for understanding how the rest of us can improve and sustain our wellbeing.

Along the way, the people who participated in my research and those in other organizations asked me to lead workshops and presentations on this science. I learned how to distill insights from research in ways people could understand and use. These were busy people whose work demanded their very best. They wanted reliable information packaged so they could take it with them. Over time, a number of those people would email or call me to say what was working for them and what wasn't. I started asking more of them what they learned from me that helped them take care of themselves. It was surprising, at first, and then deeply gratifying to know that insights from science, presented in the right way, could really help people.

In spite of what you might hear from the barrage of available self-help advice, sustaining wellbeing—your emotional, mental, and spiritual health—isn't a cleanse, a special diet, or a five-step process. We live in a world obsessed with efficiency, optimization, and instant gratification, but taking care of yourself and the people you love can be a messy, gradual process. It's an investment with spiritual and psychological returns, not financial ones. It's practice over performance: showing up every day, in whatever way you can, as you undertake the wonderful journey we call life. Helping you journey skillfully is what this book is about.

The journey metaphor is helpful for mastering the essentials of wellbeing. At the most basic level, it reminds you that wellbeing is an integral part of your life. And like life itself, wellbeing is not a destination that you reach and never leave. You age, get sick and injured. These affect your wellbeing, as do external forces, from smaller-scale challenges like flight delays and traffic jams to major life crises like a pandemic, layoff, or natural disaster. You need to know how to journey well through life's peaks and valleys. This book is meant to be a starting place to help you on this journey.

Here's an analogy to frame what this book offers. When I moved from the East Coast to Denver, I purchased a field guide to the Rocky Mountains that oriented me to the region's many trails, campgrounds, flora, and fauna. It was a great resource to begin learning about my new home environment. Initially I was interested in learning where I could do multiday backpacking trips, and the orienting knowledge I found in that guide helped me plan some great hikes. Knowing "the lay of the land" also helped me find resources I could use to learn more about specific trails I wanted to explore. At some point I will want to learn about the wildflowers and birds in my new home and I will go back to that field guide to orient me again.

This book is like that field guide. It will help you understand—perhaps for the first time—the vast territory of wellbeing and the wise practices that can help you navigate it. It will equip you with the skills you need to keep moving forward and help you map out the right path to take. And when you feel lost about what to do next, you can return to it to regain your bearings.

Essentials for Journeying Well

Years ago, when I began going on backcountry hiking trips (where you put everything you need in a backpack so you can stay off grid for a week or more), I learned there are guiding principles that are essential for hiking well: "Leave no trace" to minimize your impact on the natural environment; plan well, including preparing for potential problems; pack light, ideally carrying less than 20 percent of your body weight; and take time often to notice and appreciate the beauty of the land you are hiking through. Learning how to apply those principles improved my hikes, and I still follow them any time I head out.

A good journey also involves following guiding principles that maximize your potential to improve and sustain your wellbeing. A good way to remember these four principles is to keep this phrase in mind: *Use wise practices to step back, step easy, and step together.*

The First Principle: Journey Well with Wise Practices

A good wellbeing journey requires you to use practices you can trust—ones you can be confident will improve and sustain your wellbeing. A trustworthy wellbeing practice is wise in two ways.[3] First, it is wise because it has strong scientific evidence to support how and why it will improve or sustain your wellbeing. Research studies have uncovered the underlying mechanisms or pathways through which it works. Some of the most popular remedies are unwise because they are not based on good research.

Second, it is wise when it is personalized. This means you have chosen one that fits your beliefs, preferences, or lifestyle, instead of picking it because you happened to read about it or someone recommended it to you. There is no "one size fits all" approach to wellbeing practices. What works well for someone else might not be right for you.

A brief analogy might make my approach clearer. Boosting and maintaining physical health requires using different categories of practices—physical exercise and good nutrition are two. Medical research has provided guidelines about the physical exercise we need, and there are myriad wise ways that we can get the right amount. Among my personal favorites are hiking and high-intensity interval training. A friend of mine likes road biking. Both of us can find a wise exercise practice to maintain our physical health. Likewise, once I understand nutritional guidelines, I can select healthy foods that fit my budget, lifestyle, and personal taste.

There are dozens of wise wellbeing practices, some of which appear in this book, so there are a lot to choose from. I have organized them into eight categories—Tranquil, Receptive, Persevering, Relational, Authentic, Dedicated, Engaged, and Joyful—which I cover in chapters three through ten. Within each chapter, I describe the wellbeing needs that category can address and the science behind how its practices work. This deeper "how" knowledge will empower you to identify effective practices that fit your unique needs, goals, and lifestyle. I include examples of practices in each chapter, as well as resources in the Further Reading sections you can explore to find more practices that fit that category.

I have included a wide range of wise practices in this book. Some involve reflecting on important experiences or events. Others entail taking time for introspection to learn more about yourself and your life. Still others are built on writing, especially in longhand because research shows it engages parts of our brain that open us to deeper insights and learning. (Writing on a device appears to be less effective but still better than not writing at all.)[4] Some are best done with another person, or several people, so you can benefit from their thoughts and ideas. I also offer practices that work best when you include them regularly in your daily life, and others designed for occasional use. With so many wise practices to choose from, you can find ones that are wisest for you.

The Second Principle: Begin Your Wellbeing Journey, and Stay on Track, by Stepping Back

The remaining three principles—step back, step easy, and step together—form the basic structure of a good wellbeing journey: Begin by stepping back to see where you need to go. Then journey forward by stepping easy, whenever possible joining with other people by stepping together. Every now and then, step back to make sure you're on course. Then continue stepping easy, again stepping together whenever possible.

An interview I conducted early in my research taught me a lot about the importance of stepping back. Carin, a widely admired leader of a large religious denomination, was among the first women in her organization to be appointed a national leader. Because of her strong reputation, she received dozens of annual invitations to speak nationally and internationally at universities and conferences. A long list of highly accomplished pastors and leaders named her among their most important mentors, and each year she was asked to guide another group of rising stars.

But Carin had a problem: She was struggling with chronic stress but kept ignoring it.

I had been invited to interview Carin at her office in a historic church situated on a downtown block, around the corner from the town square. I parked in front on a cobblestone street that the town's citizens had used for more than two centuries, and walked up a sweep of marble steps through the large columns that formed the facade, framing wooden doors. When I entered, I found the atrium of the church adorned with a three-story domed ceiling, an inlaid-mosaic tile floor, and marble stairs ascending to the balcony. I followed a long, carpeted aisle that bisected a huge sanctuary with tall windows and handmade seats. The tall, ornate pulpit had hosted sermons by an impressive array of historical figures.

Carin's assistant greeted me and took me to a cozy office to wait. When Carin walked into the room, she was the embodiment of a confident and compelling leader: neat but fashionably styled gray hair, wire-rimmed glasses, beige cashmere sweater, and black slacks. She greeted me with a warm smile and gentle handshake.

I was concerned that our conversation might be formal and cover only safe, impersonal topics, but Carin immediately put me at ease with her candid and often poignant stories. When I asked how she became a pastor, she told me that as a young adult she felt a call to ministry, but had no idea how, as a woman, she could pursue that vocation beyond serving in volunteer positions—women could not be ordained as pastors in her church. Things changed in college when she heard a sermon by a woman pastor. "She was so confident and compelling. I was overwhelmed with a sense of peace and assurance," Carin told me. That experience confirmed for Carin that her call was authentic. At the time of our meeting, she was one of the most senior executives in her denomination. Carin was an accomplished pastor and talented leader at the pinnacle of her career.

When I asked questions about her current work and life, however, her narrative took a surprising turn. Carin revealed that she felt like a fraud because, as she put it, "The reality is, I am a mess." I must have looked surprised, because she added, "Yes, I work hard to hide it." When I asked her to share more, she said, "My to-do list keeps growing longer. I can't seem to get things done like I could in the past. It's harder and harder for me to focus, and I am beginning to feel like I can't keep up. Most days end with me feeling exhausted." She sat back in her chair and paused for a minute before saying, "I am not sure what is going on, why I feel this way. And I don't know how to start turning things around." She was experiencing levels of stress bordering on burnout without knowing why.

The first thing Carin needed to do was step back.

Stepping back means shifting from autopilot to awareness. It involves moving back from the flow of life to notice where things are going well for you and where you are facing challenges. A truism for most of us is that time flows past quickly, and we rarely remember the details of what happens day-to-day. We might say, "I'm stressed at work," but if asked to be specific, our answer is often incomplete. Even when we think we know what is stressing us, we are rarely confident.

Let me illustrate: Can you remember what you had for your last meal yesterday? How about a week ago? A month ago? Unless you have a set menu, you probably answered yes to the first question and no to the others. Daily life is like that. You're busy juggling a long to-do list and have little space for remembering the details of each day. Stepping back helps you take stock of where you are now and establish where you need to go next on your wellbeing journey.

At one point in our conversation, Carin mentioned an unusual habit that turned out to be helpful in our work together. She kept her schedule in a large, spiral-bound calendar. Each week occupied two pages, so there was plenty of space for the notes Carin jotted down every day, recapping each event and summarizing her experience in notations like "very productive conversation" or "what a miserable meeting."

Her calendar was a goldmine of information that she could use to step back and see what had been filling her days. There were many positive experiences, like the week she spent caring for her young grandchildren ("So much joy!"). Other positive events included coffee with friends ("With them I am just Carin, not Pastor Carin"). There was a special service celebrating retiring pastors and welcoming new ones ("Loved this service! So meaningful, so profound") and several moments with her husband ("My best friend, closest confidant, and biggest champion").

The calendar was also filled with events that were frustrating and difficult. For example, Carin had spent large chunks of time on end-of-year reports that prompted notations like "Another mountain of paperwork" and "Tons of time on a report that serves no purpose." There were meetings with struggling pastors, one of them tagged with "excruciating: he seems oblivious to the toxic effect he has on his congregation." She also traveled a lot, and notes for her most recent trips showed accumulating stress: "Tired of hotel rooms, need a good weekend with [husband] at home," "Late flight, lost bags, another exhausting trip," and "Collapsed on my bed, slept in my travel clothes."

With this information, Carin was able to step back and examine both the content and quality of her daily life. At one point she said, "I didn't realize how many burdens I was carrying. I feel better just knowing that."

Research shows that noticing and acknowledging the reality of life stressors makes them less stressful.[5] A sure way to reduce the harm of difficult, stressful, and even traumatic events is to face them directly and candidly—what clinicians call radical acceptance. A scientific truism is "that which we resist, persists." Avoiding something will only accentuate its corrosive effects. When we acknowledge the things that are worrisome, nerve-racking, or fearful in our life, we experience them as less stressful. Although facing life's challenges may not be easy, radical acceptance allows us to learn and adopt better ways of responding. Over time, radical acceptance builds inner strength so that new difficulties are less threatening. We learn to be curious about what's happening rather than worried. It is empowering, sometimes exhilarating, to be able to experience difficult events without being swamped by distress. (Chapter four will show you how to develop this skill.)

After conducting more than two thousand interviews with people like Carin, I know that her story of decreased wellbeing and an inability to pinpoint its source is common. Your story may be similar. Life comes at you fast and furious. You feel something is amiss but can't figure out exactly why. Stepping back will help you gain the clarity you need for a good start to your wellbeing journey. Empowered with this knowledge, you will be ready to step easy.

One wise way to step back so you can take a closer, more objective look at what's going on in your life is a practice called Map Your Days. I have used this practice with hundreds of people, and it gets rave reviews for how helpful it is. This is your first wise practice! It is also a foundational practice in that you can adapt it in a number of different ways. I provide several variations of this practice in the chapters ahead to illustrate how it can address other wellbeing needs.

MAP YOUR DAYS

For this practice, you will need something to write with or a place to record your thoughts.

At the end of each day, make a quick evaluation of whether it was a good or bad day. Use a smiley face, a single word like "good" or "bad," or some other quick way of recording what the day was like. Please, do not overthink. Go with your gut. Then, briefly describe one high point from that day and one low point. You decide what those are; the criteria you use are the right ones.

Write just enough so that later on you will remember what happened. You will likely be able to complete this entire process in five minutes or less.

Do this each day for at least two weeks, more if you can. Then, take a look back. Note the high points on your good days and look for patterns among them. What kinds of things made the day a good one? Looking for common themes will provide you with insights about the things that make your days positive.

Next, shift to the bad days and look for patterns in the low points. Take time to recall what happened on each one. Looking deeper into those days will provide insights about what makes days stressful, challenging, or difficult. The high points on bad days may also help you discover things that can make even a tough day a little better.

End by comparing the low points from your good and bad days. If you see common patterns, return to the good days to see what might have helped you overcome or deal well with those low points.

Many of the people who have used this practice found it helpful to review their map with someone who knows them well. Significant others can offer beneficial insights and ideas, and may help you spot things you missed.

The wellbeing assessment at the end of chapter two is another good way to step back and identify where you can improve your wellbeing. Better still, use both the assessment and Map Your Days to get a more comprehensive perspective on where you are in your journey.

The Third Principle: Sustain Your Journey by Stepping Easy

People often tell me they think improving their wellbeing will require big changes, and they don't have the time or energy to make them. But big changes are almost never the best choice. This is partly because they do require a lot of time and energy, but also because big changes often have unintended effects that cause more problems. A better choice is to do little things often enough to create big changes. I call this stepping easy. Let me illustrate.

The achievement gap experienced by students who are members of ethnic, racial, or socioeconomic minorities is well documented.[6] These students earn lower grades than their majority-group peers, and their grades decline each year, making it more likely that they will drop out. Many explanations have long been offered for this gap, including poverty, immigration status, parenting practices, and limited English literacy. The traditional approach to remedying these situations was putting students in "special needs" classes, offering rewards for good performance, and, sometimes, using detention or temporary suspension for students who underperformed.

A group of researchers led by psychologist David Sherman at the University of California, Santa Barbara, had another idea: What if the gap was caused by stresses stemming from being a member of a negatively stereotyped group?[7] Adolescence is a crucial developmental period when young people are struggling with existential questions like: Do I have any talents or skills? Am I a person of value? Am I smart? These researchers hypothesized that the psychological burdens of negative stereotypes might undermine at-risk students' sense of personal value and academic competency. They also thought these effects might accumulate over time and cause persistent declines in academic performance. Early academic failures, such as a poor grade, could reinforce the burdens—"Maybe I *am not* smart enough for school"—creating a growing snowball of declining self-worth and performance.

These scientists thought a simple practice called values affirmations might help alleviate the negative effects of being stereotyped. A common values affirmation practice is to write for ten minutes about one of your core life values such as a commitment to social justice, a belief in a loving God, or a passion for sports. You write about what it is and why it matters to you, then write for ten minutes about a time you did something that lived out or honored that value.

Values affirmation practices work by creating a psychological timeout, a chance to regain perspective on what matters in life. In doing so, they remind people of something they value deeply, which can be a source of strength during adversity. Researchers hypothesized that this might broaden students' self-worth by reinforcing that their personal value is more than the negative judgments of other people, which, in turn, could ameliorate their psychological burdens.

Sherman and his colleagues conducted two studies to test their idea. The first study involved 196 at-risk middle school boys and girls, whom they divided into two groups. The first was a control group that would go about school in the usual way. The second group would do a values affirmation exercise before the first week of the new school year. Importantly, teachers had no idea which students were part of the study, so any results would be free from their influence.

The results were remarkable. After that first year, the control group students showed the typical decline in academic performance, but the students who had done the simple twenty-minute values affirmation practice did not. Even more remarkable, this pattern continued for two more years despite the students having done the values affirmation practice only once. The performance of the control group continued to decline, while the values-affirmed students continued to perform well, nearly on par with majority students. Because the study ended after year three, we don't know if the positive outcomes persisted, but the pattern suggests that they did.

The second study was done with a group of two hundred seventh graders. As in the first study, the students were divided into two groups. Half did the values affirmation practice before the first week of school. The other half were the control group and went through the typical school entry process. Both groups answered questions about their self-worth and self-confidence. The researchers then gathered data about the students' academic performance, self-worth, and self-confidence during each of the following three years. The performance of the control group followed the typical declining pattern each successive year, while the performance of the values-affirmed students increased. The self-worth and self-confidence of the control group students also declined year after year, while the values-affirmed students reported increases in both. Imagine what might have happened if the students had done the values affirmation practice each year!

This easy, wise practice that took only twenty minutes to do overcame social stereotype threats, changed students' sense of self-worth, and increased their academic performance for at least three years.

Stepping easy reflects the scientific insight that, with rare exceptions, your wellbeing improves or declines through the buildup of small, often imperceptible changes. No one burns out all at once, for example. Burnout creeps up through an accumulation of difficult days, stressful events, and perhaps a few bad experiences. This is why almost no one sees it coming. The same is true for most of your wellbeing-related problems. They have built up over time, and you probably didn't notice them until they became conspicuous. If you are stressed out, it is not because of the last tough day you had. Like Carin, your stress is the result of an accumulation of burdensome days and difficult interactions. In the same way, boosting your wellbeing usually requires doing little things often enough that they create big improvements.

Most of the wise practices I share in this book take only a few minutes and can slip into even a busy schedule. They are easy and will fit into the normal flow of your day, such as when you are stopped at a red light, commuting on the bus or train, or brushing your teeth. Yet they can create significant improvements in your wellbeing.

All of the practices in this book are wise ways to step easy. They work best when you do them routinely and faithfully. Stepping easy with wise practices is similar to physical exercises like weight training. You build strength by getting in enough repetitions, spread out over weeks and months. While muscles grow during each day of exercise, you can only see those changes when you look back at where you started and compare that to where you are now. Even so, positive change happens each time you practice.

Most days, the shifts in your wellbeing will be small and subtle. Sometimes, you will experience profound changes, such as a moment of deep insight, a transformation in your self-understanding, or a more positive dynamic in your spiritual life. But usually, the best way to see improvements in your wellbeing is to step back and compare where you are now to where you started. Repeating the wellbeing assessment in chapter two every few months is a good way to create wellbeing milestones to track your progress.

While easy steps won't fix your wellbeing needs immediately—there are no quick fixes—practicing regularly will lead to lasting and positive change. And since easy steps fit nicely into your days, you will be able to find one you can start right away.

The Fourth Principle: Journey with Good Companions by Stepping Together

Stepping together, the fourth principle, reminds us that there are tight links between our wellbeing and the wellbeing of the people in our lives. The rugged individualism we prize so much in America tells us that we are masters of our own destinies. If things are going badly for you, that norm tells you to pull yourself up by your bootstraps. But the truth is much more complicated: Other people are also pulling and pushing on your boots.

A long-term study of the residents of Framingham, Massachusetts, provides hard evidence that our wellbeing is socially embedded.[8] Since the study's inception in 1948, three generations of Framingham citizens have volunteered to participate in what has become one of the largest, longest, and most important health and wellbeing studies ever conducted. The National Institutes of Health call the Framingham Heart Study the "crown jewel of epidemiology."

The origins of the study are linked to the 1945 death of President Franklin D. Roosevelt at age sixty-three from hypertensive heart disease. In 1948, in response to a groundswell of concern, Congress passed the National Heart Act, which included funds for what would become the Framingham Heart Study. Massachusetts was selected because of the positive response of local physicians, and Framingham was selected both because of its proximity to Harvard Medical School and because about two thousand of its residents had participated in a tuberculosis study twenty-five years earlier. A young physician, Gilcin Meadors, was appointed the study's first director. When he and his assistants began recruiting participants, Framingham residents responded enthusiastically: 5,209 of the approximately 10,000 adults volunteered. This was not a simple effort. Participants were poked, prodded, and intensely scrutinized. They underwent extensive physical examinations, gave blood samples for laboratory tests, and answered long surveys about their lifestyle and medical history. And they endured this year after year.

The study has produced an astounding number of groundbreaking discoveries. Among the first breakthroughs was identifying the key risk factors for cardiovascular disease, including the effects of cholesterol, high blood pressure, smoking, and obesity. Framingham research has also led to discoveries about other health conditions including osteoporosis, dementia, diabetes, Parkinson's disease, and cancer.

One of the important things about this study, which is still ongoing today, is that it involves a cohort of people living in the same community. This has allowed researchers to dig deep into the social causes of wellbeing. And because the participants live in the same place, researchers have been able to separate the impact of social factors from environmental conditions. They found that social causes matter a lot more. Even more remarkable, as sociologists Nicholas Christakis and James Fowler describe it in their book *Connected: The Surprising Power of Our Social Networks and How They Shape Our Lives*, the Framingham study shows that it's not just your family and friends that have a significant impact on your wellbeing; it is also your friends' friends' friends.[9] This is an extremely important discovery. It means that, like the ecosystems we see in the natural world, the web of social connections we are embedded in—at home, at work, in neighborhoods, and in communities—has profound consequences for our health and wellbeing.

For example, Framingham researchers discovered that if individuals in your social ecosystem are obese, your chances of becoming obese increase significantly. If your spouse becomes obese, the likelihood that you will become obese increases 37 percent. If a friend becomes obese, your chances nearly triple. People more distant in your ecosystem matter too. As Christakis and Fowler write, "You may not know him personally, but your friend's husband's coworker can make you fat. And your sister's friend's boyfriend can make you thin."[10]

Further, as Christakis and Fowler describe, the study revealed that your chances of becoming depressed double if a friend becomes depressed, and quadruple if a next-door neighbor does. Happily, happiness also spreads among the people in your wellbeing ecosystems. You are 75 percent more likely to become happy if you have a happy friend. Even a happy neighbor a mile away boosts your chances 25 percent.

Various other studies now confirm the impact of wellbeing ecosystems. For example, researchers have documented that burnout spreads among coworkers, including between bosses and their subordinates.[11] In a study of over 1,200 teachers working at 26 different schools, researchers found that burnout spread among colleagues who had daily interactions.[12] More surprisingly, this ecosystem effect lasted two years, meaning that if you worked with a burned-out teacher two years ago, you're more likely to burn out today.

A massive twenty-year study of more than 680,000 people shows our social connections matter even when we are never face-to-face with other people. This study showed that happiness and depression can spread through social media.[13] A similar study found that anxiety during the pandemic spread through online networks.[14] In other words, simply reading about or seeing pictures of what people in your ecosystem are doing, feeling, and thinking can affect your wellbeing.

Here's a quick way for you to visualize the potential size of your ecosystem. Think of twenty people you are close to—a partner, family members, friends, neighbors, and coworkers. Now, imagine that each of those twenty people also has twenty close connections. This places you in the middle of an ecosystem of as many as eight thousand people who, for better and for worse, can shape your wellbeing.

In a rare instance of near universal agreement, scientists are adamant that wellbeing isn't an individual quest, a solo climb to the top, a destination you reach alone. Wellbeing is embedded in the ties that bind and the spaces that hold us together. It is knitted into the social threads that weave us to others. When we neglect or ignore those threads, we not only jeopardize our wellbeing, but we also may imperil the people we are connected to.

While wise practices can strengthen our social connections, stepping together is more than something we do occasionally. It is part of the underlying rhythm of how we live our days, a way of moving through life in harmony with other people, the world, and something infinitely beyond. It shows up in the ways we interact with people we see regularly—family, friends, acquaintances, coworkers—and in the ways we treat people we may see only once. It happens in moments of synchronicity when we feel deeply connected to another person and in the brief exchanges we have with a customer service agent. Stepping together happens in raucous parties where we celebrate with significant others and the quiet sharing when we read to a child. And it happens most poignantly when we care for someone who is experiencing injury, illness, or loss, or when we are the beneficiary of that kind of care. At its core, stepping together is the interplay of giving and receiving, of caring and being cared for, of loving and being loved.

Good relationships and strong social support are among the most important determinants of sustained wellbeing. You need these kinds of relationships in all of the important areas of your life. The principle of stepping together reminds you that finding and traveling with good companions is an essential part of a healthy wellbeing journey. It also reminds you to be intentional about finding wise ways to respect, support, love, and care for others. Throughout this book I offer examples of practices that are also wise ways to step together. You may have some of your own favorites, and if you do, keep using them.

Taking Your First Step

It's time to begin your wellbeing journey. The best way to start is by stepping back to identify your wellbeing needs and goals. Chapter two will equip you with the knowledge and tools you need to decide where you want to journey next. Then, journey forward by stepping easy and, whenever possible, journey with good companions by stepping together. From time to time, step back to see the progress you've made and figure out where to go next. Then journey forward again by stepping easy and stepping together.

As I mentioned, all of the practices I share are good ways to step easy. They are all based on solid research, so they are also wise in the first sense. They can also be wise in the second sense if they fit your beliefs, preferences, or lifestyle. Where practices are not just stepping easy, but also ways to step back or step together, I have indicated this with these icons.

There's an old aphorism that any journey begins with the first step, and I appreciate the deeper meaning it conveys. You can't take the entire journey all at once. But the first step can be one of the hardest ones to take. That's where you are now, ready to take that first step. Chapter two will help you figure out the right first step and empower you to take it with confidence.

CHAPTER TWO

Wellbeing

What It Is and How You Are Doing

If I asked you to describe what wellbeing is, what would you say? I've asked hundreds of people that question, and while most said they weren't sure, almost everyone felt that happiness was a key part of it. They are in good company. As historian Darrin McMahon notes, throughout history, happiness has been equated with the most perfect human state.[1] The Founders of the United States held similar beliefs; the Declaration of Independence names "the pursuit of happiness" as one of the three inalienable human rights. But, therein lies the challenge, as Benjamin Franklin remarked: "[The Declaration] only gives you the right to pursue happiness. You have to catch it yourself."[2]

Americans seem to have taken that challenge seriously. About a century after the signing of the Declaration, the great American psychologist and philosopher William James observed that "how to gain, how to keep, how to recover happiness, is in fact for most men at all times the secret motive of all they do, and of all they are willing to endure."[3] That secret motive has persisted into modern times, so much so that some cultural critics have argued that "Americans are obsessed with happiness."[4] One critic even asserted that the pursuit of happiness "has undermined America."[5]

Americans aren't alone in this preoccupation: Happiness is now a major concern around the world. In 2012 the United Nations General Assembly declared March 20 the International Day of Happiness to encourage member states to strive toward "a more inclusive, equitable and balanced approach to economic growth that promotes the happiness and wellbeing of all peoples." Since then, a group of researchers has assessed the happiness of people from 130 countries each year and published the results in the World Happiness Report.[6] Using a simple but accurate measure called Cantril's Ladder, they collect information from at least three thousand people in each country, then average their answers to arrive at a nation's happiness score.

You can use it to measure your own happiness right now. Imagine a ladder with eleven rungs. The lowest rung, numbered zero, represents what, for you, would be the worst possible life and the greatest possible unhappiness. The top rung, numbered ten, represents what, for you, would be the best possible life and the greatest possible happiness. Which rung are you standing on right now? How happy are you?

In the 2024 report, Finland was the happiest country, with an average ladder score of 7.74. Afghans were standing on the lowest rung with an average of 1.72. People in the United States placed themselves at 6.72, but this is nearly a full rung lower than in 2023. Happiness levels in Mexico (6.68), the United Kingdom (6.75), and France (6.61) did not change significantly over that time.

But is happiness really essential for wellbeing?

Answering that question is what this chapter is about. We will explore a science-based model of wellbeing to give you a solid understanding you can count on. Using that model, along with the short assessment I provide, you will be able to evaluate your own.

Here's a metaphor to get us started: At its most basic level, we can define health as the physical energy, muscular strength and endurance, and brain functionality you need to live a full and active life. We can go a step deeper and describe the dimensions—cardiovascular, neurological, and musculoskeletal—that are integral to creating physical health. We would also want to emphasize that these dimensions are tightly linked and affect one another. For example, gastrointestinal health is essential for sustaining your muscles, bones, heart, and other organs, and it is also the source of the physical energy that powers your body.

We can also start with a very basic definition of wellbeing: the emotional stability, mental acuity, and spiritual grounding you need to live each day fully and well. We can then explore the dimensions that are integral for creating wellbeing: happiness, resilience, connectedness, self-integrity, and meaning.

Notice how, like the different elements of health, they are tightly linked. As one dimension increases, it tends to increase the others as well. Unfortunately, the reverse is also true: When one becomes particularly low, it tends to drag down the others. This means that we need to pay attention to all five dimensions, noticing and addressing any that are dipping down significantly. Sure, you can ignore the grind of stressful days (low happiness), or push on while lonely in life (low connectedness), or fill your days with pursuits that are not very important

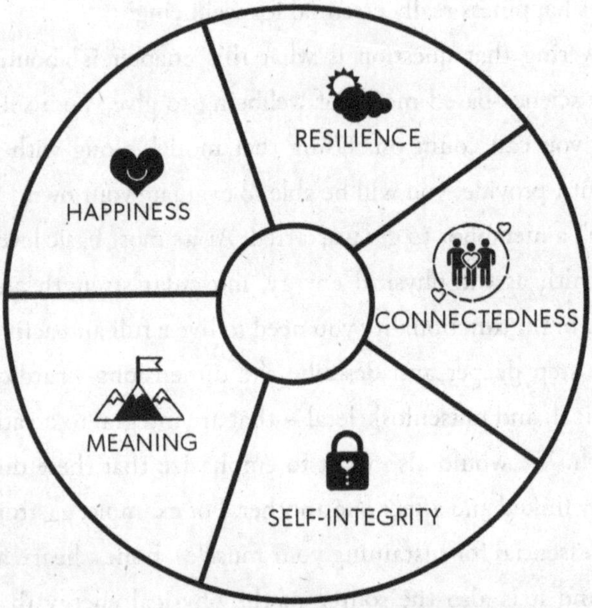

to you (low meaning), but over time those choices will likely deplete your wellbeing in every dimension.

You will likely experience lower wellbeing when you are ill or injured, and likewise you will feel physically tired and be more prone to illness during periods of high stress or when your resilience is low. But—and this is important—you can still maintain high wellbeing over time even when you experience physical health challenges. Like me, you may know people with chronic health issues like early-onset Parkinson's disease, persistent back pain, or cancer who are still very happy and resilient, have deeply meaningful lives and caring relationships, and have a strong sense of self-worth. Unfortunately, I also know people who are very healthy, but are leading unhappy, meaningless, lonely lives. So, while health and wellbeing are related to some extent, they are not locked together permanently.

Let's explore the dimensions of wellbeing by starting with the important but confusing topic of happiness.

Happiness: The Quality of Your Daily Life

People who knew University of Illinois Professor Ed Diener said he was one of the nicest, kindest, and happiest people they ever met. He reminded me of Mister Rogers: always smiling, always cheerful, and always thinking about other people.

Professor Diener was also a prolific scholar who invented happiness research in the 1980s. He established that happiness is a combination of three factors: feeling many positive moods and emotions, feeling few negative moods and emotions, and having a generally positive evaluation of the quality of your life (Cantril's Ladder again). Researchers use the term "affect" in place of "moods" or "emotions," so happiness = positive affect + life satisfaction – negative affect.

Positive affect comes in many different forms: peacefulness, contentment, compassion, cheerfulness, curiosity, pride, interest, generosity, enthusiasm, wonder, love, and joy. Similarly, there are many kinds of negative affect, including boredom, irritation, frustration, worry, fear, anger, grief, envy, and sadness. What matters for happiness is the pattern of daily moods and emotions you experience over time.

A rough rule of thumb is that we should have about four positive affect experiences for every negative one. To maintain wellbeing, we want this ratio to be the typical pattern we experience over the course of days, weeks, and months. This is a best estimate, so think of it as a guideline, not a hard-and-fast rule.[7] We all have bad days and weeks as we experience difficulties and challenges in life, and times like those are, understandably, not going to be very happy. But they do not doom us to perpetual unhappiness.

We also need to understand that the *kinds* of positive and negative affect we experience matter. Pleasure seeking does not build happiness, and neither does artificially inducing positive feelings by, for example, using alcohol or drugs. In fact, over time both of these happiness pursuits create unhappiness.

Experiencing mostly positive affect has some really important benefits. Diener and his colleagues reviewed 225 happiness studies and concluded as follows:

> Numerous studies show that happy individuals are successful across multiple life domains, including marriage, friendship, income, work performance, and health . . . [T]he happiness–success link exists not only because success makes people happy, but also because positive affect engenders success . . . Furthermore, the evidence suggests that positive affect—the hallmark of wellbeing—may be the cause of many of the desirable characteristics, resources, and successes correlated with happiness.[8]

Among these desirable outcomes are better physical health, higher self-confidence, less conflict in life, a greater propensity to be helpful to others, better decision-making, higher performance in almost any endeavor, greater creativity, and increased capacity to form and sustain positive relationships.[9]

Flip that four-to-one ratio around and you get the scientific description of chronic stress. Chronic stress occurs when acute stress—negative affect and troublesome thought—has accumulated over days or weeks. It can lead to cardiovascular disease, increased susceptibility to infections of many kinds, depression, and burnout, among other health and wellbeing challenges.[10] It wears us down and saps our resilience (the second dimension of wellbeing).

One thing that makes happiness elusive is that when today becomes yesterday, we tend to forget the details of what made our days either good or bad. Recall how you responded to the "remember what you ate" question in the previous chapter. Again, the key is to find ways to have more good days.

Positive evaluations of your life, the third element of happiness, is how you summarize the quality of your day-to-day experiences (Cantril's Ladder again). Do you think things are going well for you? Is your life moving in the right direction? Whether you realize it or not, you are forming these life satisfaction evaluations each day. So, for example, if you have had a lot of good days, you are likely to feel very satisfied with your life. The reverse is also true: If you have experienced an accumulation of difficult days, you will likely have lower life satisfaction.

The key insight from research is that we need our typical day-to-day experience to be tipped toward happiness. Science does not advocate for us to try to eliminate all unhappy feelings; rather, it alerts us to pay attention to the negative feelings we experience and find ways to respond well to them. Ignoring stress, for example, will not work. The better approach is to reduce or eliminate sources of stress when we can and learn how to cope effectively with the stress we cannot stop.

Tranquil practices (chapter three) and joyful practices (chapter ten) will help you boost and sustain happiness. Receptive practices (chapter four) and persevering practices (chapter five) will help you create a less stressful pattern to your daily life.

Resilience: Your Capacity to Cope, Adapt, and Grow

Kristie always felt drawn to humanitarian work. She grew up in a family where volunteering at community outreach programs was a weekly commitment. She remembers toddling around soup kitchens with her parents, and during her elementary school years, she joined her church's ministry that served unhoused people. That pattern of commitment to social service grew even stronger in high school and culminated in her decision to join an international aid organization after college.

Fast-forward to when I met Kristie. She was in her twentieth year of humanitarian work, having worked in more than a dozen countries and now the senior leader in charge of programs serving several thousand people in Southeast Asia. She was also part of her organization's emergency response team, a select group of people who fly into disaster areas during a crisis. Over her tenure, Kristie had been among the first people on the ground in response to more than a dozen natural disasters.

What stood out to me about Kristie was her ability to effectively navigate the highs and lows of humanitarian work for so many years. She admitted that sometimes the difficulties seemed to pile up, but she'd learned to step back regularly and check in on her wellbeing. She had a collection of wise wellbeing practices she used every day. She'd learned how to set boundaries so work would not encroach into her family and personal time, she worked with a spiritual director to keep tabs on what she calls her "spiritual wellspring," and she had a daily contemplative practice.

During our first meeting, Kristie shared that she was preparing to move to a new post in Africa to take on an even larger leadership role. Her youngest child would start college in the United States soon, and her husband's work required that he stay in their current location, so they would be adjusting to a long-distance relationship. As she put it, "I no longer have the unstoppable energy of youth. I am not just getting older, I *am* older, and to keep doing this work I have to make adjustments." She was facing a series of changes that could compromise her wellbeing.

When I met with Kristie eighteen months later, she was energetic, vibrant, and inspired by her new work. Her daughter's first year of college had gone very well and her relationship with her husband was stronger than ever. She loved her new work and the programs she was leading were exceeding expectations. She said she was "flourishing."

Kristie is able to roll so well with the highs and lows of life and work because she is resilient.

Resilience comprises your capacity to deal well with the vicissitudes of daily life, as well as your capacity to adapt and grow as the world around you changes.[11] Resilient people may experience temporary declines in their overall wellbeing, but because they recover quickly, they are also able to adjust to changing life situations (e.g., the birth of a child, moving to a new home, starting a new job), and to adversity and crisis (e.g., job loss, a serious health challenge, the death of a loved one).

Resilience has two core elements: psychological flexibility and adaptive coping. Psychological flexibility encompasses self-awareness and self-reflectivity. Self-awareness is the capacity to pay attention to and recognize what is happening inside you as challenging or troublesome things happen outside you. We are often unaware of why we do the things we do. We may come up with explanations for our behaviors, but a big chunk of it is beyond our conscious awareness. People with high self-awareness avoid this; they are more cognizant of the reasons behind their actions. They are aware of thoughts like "I am feeling this particular mood or emotion," "I am thinking about this issue," or "I responded to that person in this specific way." When we describe someone as being "a bull in a china shop," we are describing someone with little to no self-awareness. Self-awareness is not self-consciousness, that overly sensitive, uncomfortable form of self-focus many of us experienced as teenagers. It is being conscious of your thoughts and feelings without being entangled or obsessed with them.

Self-reflectivity is the capacity to examine your thoughts, feelings, and behaviors, especially in terms of whether or not they are appropriate, good, helpful, or otherwise positive for yourself and others. Self-awareness provides information about what is happening inside you, and through self-reflectivity you gain an understanding of why you are thinking, feeling, or acting in certain ways. It is not ruminating about yourself, working each thought or feeling into a knotty ball of hyper self-criticism; it is the capacity to gain insights into those experiences and their likely causes.

Reinhold Niebuhr's famous "Serenity Prayer" is a masterful summary of adaptive coping, the second core element of resilience: "God, give us grace to accept with serenity the things that cannot be changed / Courage to change the things which should be changed / and the Wisdom to distinguish the one from the other." Once self-awareness and self-reflectivity have provided the information about what is happening in and around you, adaptive coping is the capacity to respond effectively to that information. It includes both your ability to change the world around you when you can (e.g., finding a less stressful job, rescheduling your day to make time to relax, putting your phone in a locked drawer to prevent checking your social media accounts) and your ability to adapt and change yourself (e.g., giving up a bad habit, learning how to manage worrisome thoughts, finding better ways to interact with a difficult person). And, as Niebuhr's prayer emphasizes, adaptive coping also encompasses your ability to distinguish when you should try to change the world around you, when you should change, and when you have to adjust to things as they are.

There are strong connections between happiness and resilience. If you have a series of bad days, you will use a lot of your resilience reserves. You can get stretched so thin that even simple problems might seem insurmountable. Left unaddressed, this combination of chronic stress and low resilience can create serious problems. It's important to keep your resilience capacities as strong as possible, especially when daily life gets rocky.

Receptive practices (chapter four) and persevering practices (chapter five) will help you learn how to maintain resilience even when daily life is difficult.

Connectedness: Love, Care, and Social Relationships

When I interviewed Hillary, Jill, and Tina, they were all field managers at an international humanitarian organization. Each worked in a hardship post and had experience working in field camps in several countries. At the time I spoke with them, they were working in different locations, separated by distance and time zones. Hillary and Jill had recently had their first children, and both were experiencing the challenges of managing family and work. When I asked about their support group, all three spoke first about their partners and the incredible support they provided. And quickly thereafter, they spoke about each other.

Hillary said:

> There's two people, and I just feel like my friendships with them are being strengthened each time I see or talk with them. I can share a little bit more about myself as a person and as a professional with them. Jill would be the closest person that if I needed something, I would call her and say, "Oh my gosh, I just need to talk about this," and she listens. When we talk or see each other, we just dive, I just feel like we can both be very honest with each other about our struggles or our joys. Tina is so fun and she's always positive so whenever I talk to her, I'm usually laughing the whole time and we're talking about memories or whatever else is happening in our lives at the moment. That's what cements our friendship.

All three friends described the joys and sorrows of working in overseas posts. And while working with marginalized and victimized people is deeply meaningful, it can also be very difficult and, at times, even traumatic. Jill shared that she leans on Hillary and Tina during those difficult moments: "I can talk to them on the phone and be like, 'They just pulled a body out in front of me a couple of hours ago, people are crying. I'm just so tired.' They get it, they get how emotionally tiring it is. And then at other times, we laugh about the funny things going on in our lives. And sometimes, we just sit on the phone and cry together."

As in many organizations, the remnants of patriarchy are still prevalent in humanitarian agencies, and women often have to work harder to gain the respect of their colleagues. Jill described the ways this trio helps each other navigate these challenges: "Something I really appreciate . . . is we are highlighting each other's successes in front of people who may not know about them. We call it out. When [Hillary and Tina] name something I have done, I feel really supported. It feels good and it feels encouraging."

I asked what keeps their friendship strong, and Tina described it this way: "We know we can trust each other. We all know why we're here and why we're doing this work—like me, they really care. So, we have this deep bond around what we care about. That's why I can trust them, trust their hearts. That's why I know I can depend on them."

Their friendship illustrates the central role connectedness plays in wellbeing.

Connectedness is the quality of the relationships in one's life. We are social beings; we cannot live or thrive without strong and positive social connections. Relationships with others have an immense impact on our physical health and wellbeing. We need to feel loved and cared for by family and friends, respected and valued by our colleagues at work and in other major life activities, and properly supported in all the situations where we give our time and effort. A blue-ribbon panel of medical and social scientists appointed to review the importance of connectedness concluded:

Extensive scientific findings from a variety of disciplines, including epidemiology, neuroscience, medicine, psychology, and sociology, converge on the same conclusion: social connection is a significant predictor of longevity and better physical, cognitive, and mental health, while social isolation and loneliness are significant predictors of premature death and poor health. In fact, the benefits of social connection extend beyond health-related outcomes. They influence an individual's educational attainment, workplace satisfaction, economic prosperity, and overall feelings of wellbeing and life fulfillment.[14]

Even though most of us interact with people nearly every day, many of us lack the social support we need. Dr. Vivek Murthy, the former US surgeon general, declared there is an epidemic of loneliness in America: One in two adults in the United States reported experiencing social isolation.[15]

The most important social connections are those in which we experience care, compassion, and acceptance. Positive connectedness means we feel respected for who we are and affirmed and validated for our strengths and talents, as well as for our idiosyncrasies, our uniqueness, and even our oddities. I can be very scatterbrained and often poorly organized. In conversations, I often venture off to explore new ideas. The upside of this is that I am creative. The downside is that I can derail conversations. Nevertheless, I know my family and friends accept and respect me. The care they show me helps me harness my creativity in more focused and positive ways.

Positive relationships provide the psychological and social resources we need to get through life's most difficult challenges. Researchers

Brooke Feeney and Nancy Collins have found two kinds of social support to be essential for positive relationships: acting as a source of strength and as a relational catalyst.[16] Acting as a source of strength involves creating a safe refuge during times of adversity; providing emotional support, safety, and protection; and relieving the burdens a valued other experiences. Acting as a relational catalyst involves encouraging someone to fully embrace life's opportunities for growth. This includes, for example, validating and expressing enthusiasm for their goals and aspirations, encouraging them to embrace challenges, and emphasizing the potential benefits of these opportunities.

Chapter six, on relational practices, provides scientific insights that show how simple, everyday practices keep relationships strong, help repair them when they break down, and create ways for us to build new positive connections.

Self-Integrity: Your Identity and Sense of Self-Worth

I met Naomi on a weekday morning. She was serving as an associate pastor for a large church in a college town. We met in a beautiful sanctuary and, from the very beginning of our conversation, Naomi exuded positivity and warmth. She spoke openly and easily about her ministry experiences. Her relaxed professionalism conveyed self-confidence.

Naomi said she "grew up with a really clear sense of vocation. My mother is a church worker and my grandfather is a pastor. My father is a scientist, with a theological wonder at the universe, and a belief of doing what you were equipped for, in ways that God can use your gifts in the world. I knew whatever I did was going to be for the good of the world because of God's love . . . I was shaped to be a pastor. I'm not sure I could be anybody else if I tried."

Naomi's first position after seminary was as a solo pastor of a small rural church. She said that position created a lot of opportunities for professional growth, and for that she was grateful. Naomi married during her time there. After two years, she was asked to serve as an assistant to an older, male senior pastor. He had a top-down leadership style and made all of the ministry decisions. Naomi had both of her children during that time, and she described many patronizing interactions where he questioned her ability to manage a family and be a pastor. Their styles of ministry were as different as the generations into which they were born. For example, the senior pastor remained aloof from the congregation while she worked hard to form relationships with church members. When he abruptly retired a couple of years later, Naomi went from being an assistant to being the lead minister.

Naomi became the first female senior pastor at this church. Being thrust into an unanticipated role required her to develop new skills and capabilities very quickly. It turned out to be a period of growth for both Naomi and the congregation. She was honest about the challenges and rewards of personal and professional change during that time. When I spoke with her, she was five years into this new role. Reflecting on what she learned about herself, she said, "The last five years have been about confidence in leadership." She described herself as a shy person who "plays a mean second fiddle," but she learned she can "serve with skill and grace in a primary leadership role." Naomi said that an important part of her growth was learning to be honest with herself about who she is. She'd learned about the skills and talents she has, and the ones she lacks. She was aware of what she called her "darker nature," the tendencies and impulses she has to manage. Most of all, Naomi said she now felt "comfortable in my own skin, comfortable to be myself in ways that are also good for the congregation and church staff."

Naomi is an example of someone who has strong self-integrity.

Self-integrity, the fourth building block of wellbeing, is having a balanced, secure, and positive identity. People who have self-integrity understand and affirm the knowledge, skills, and abilities they possess and know how to put them to productive use. They also acknowledge their weaknesses, negative tendencies, and deficiencies. Researchers call this "authenticity": when people know themselves well and, therefore, like Naomi, are comfortable in their own skin.

Importantly, self-integrity is independent of comparisons with other people. As two leading researchers of self-integrity—Stanford University psychologist Geoffrey Cohen and David Sherman, his University of California, Santa Barbara, colleague—emphasize, "It is not to be superior or excellent, but to be 'good enough.'"[12] Unfortunately, our culture creates constant pressures to compare ourselves to other people. We face it in nearly every social context we experience: at work, in the gym, at events at our kids' school, even at church or in the grocery store. Social media is especially rife with prompts to measure yourself against the people in your network. Princeton psychologist Susan Fiske, an expert on social comparison, writes that "comparison compels people, even as it stresses, depresses, and divides us. Comparison is only natural, but the collateral damage reveals envy upward and scorn downward, and these emotions . . . poison people and their relationships."[13] Having self-integrity means feeling good about yourself without regard to how you stack up against others.

Authentic practices (chapter seven) strengthen and sustain self-integrity. Relational practices (chapter six) and dedicated practices (chapter eight) also help you and the people in your life find a secure and stable sense of self-worth.

Meaning: Significance, Certitude, Purpose, and Spirituality

When I first met Karl, he looked more like a rumpled nerd than a senior leader of a large international humanitarian organization responsible for more than a thousand programs throughout the Middle East and Africa. Small in stature, balding, and disheveled in his khaki pants and white button-down shirt, he was so unassuming that I initially looked past him as I scanned the hotel lobby where we planned to meet. Karl waved vigorously to catch my attention, and that was my first exposure to his boundless energy and enthusiasm. I soon learned that talking with Karl was usually an exciting and somewhat chaotic adventure. He spoke with a rapid, staccato pace I initially found hard to keep up with.

Karl had spent more than three decades in the humanitarian field. He had worked in the most difficult and dangerous contexts, including posts in areas with active hostilities and those devastated by natural disasters. He was a highly respected leader in charge of the largest and most complex programs, including major famine relief efforts and refugee projects serving thousands of displaced individuals. Karl's subordinates described him as a deeply caring, wise, and astute leader. One of his senior associates said, "There is no problem he can't solve and no situation so complex he can't find a way forward. I'm sure he has ten thousand things on his to-do list, but whenever I talk to him it seems like he has all the time in the world. I don't know how he can do so much and remain so positive."

I collaborated with Karl for over a decade during my research on the wellbeing of humanitarian workers, but one incident stands out. We were in a meeting with a group of US graduate students interested in humanitarian work. Karl was invited to participate with senior leaders from other organizations to share their experiences about working in that sector. During the meeting, Rachel Carson was offered as a model of someone whose commitment to helping others was exemplary. Her book *Silent Spring* is credited with launching the global environmental movement. The other senior leaders affirmed Carson as a consummate humanitarian.

Karl seemed concerned. During a pause in the conversation, he stood up and said, "Rachel Carson's work also contributed to the deaths of thousands of people." The group looked at Karl with dismay. Speaking with emotion, he continued, "The bans on DDT that resulted from her book have created an explosion in mosquito-borne diseases. Malaria. Elephantiasis. Dengue fever. These diseases have caused immense suffering, especially among the most vulnerable people in the world. She is remembered as a hero, but the consequences of her work have also been devastating."

Several of the students protested that, without those bans, hundreds of animal species would be extinct. Karl countered with a poignant statement, "What is more valuable to you: human lives or the lives of animals? If you follow a path into humanitarian work, there will be times you will have to make difficult moral choices. Humanitarian work is immensely important and it can be profoundly rewarding. But you have to know where you stand. Otherwise, you may find yourself in moral quandaries that will crush your spirit for this work."

A few months ago, I heard from Karl that he had "retired," which for him meant helping others through volunteer engagements. He was helping male prison inmates transition back into civilian life and serving at a local soup kitchen, and was looking for even more opportunities to "give back," which made me smile because I see Karl's entire adult life as a gift to help others. He was happy and thriving, feeling a renewed joy for life and for his work.

Karl's passion and commitment to serving others, and his ability to navigate the rough moral terrain it sometimes requires, are outcomes of his strong sense of meaning.

The idea that meaning is important for human flourishing has very ancient roots, going back at least to the ancient Greeks. Aristotle was the first person to formally study this dimension of wellbeing, which he referred to as "eudaemonia." The Greek *daimon* refers to our spirit or deepest state of being, and the prefix *eu-* means good, so eudaemonia is having a good indwelling spirit. Researchers have expanded upon these ideas, exploring the characteristics of experiencing meaning in life, and finding that it is strongly linked to health and wellbeing.[17]

Consensus is growing among scholars that experiencing meaning in life arises from three constituents: a belief that there is inherent value in life and that your own life has value and importance (significance); a sense that you are able to contribute to important life aspirations (purpose); and an understanding of what life is truly about that makes existence comprehensible, especially in the face of life's uncertainties and difficulties (certitude).[18] For many people, an important fourth element is experiencing a connection with something sacred that is "greater than and more important than" themselves, something that is often understood to be divine, or in some way transcendent to or "beyond" our normal, everyday material world (spirituality).[19]

Significance is a belief that life itself has inherent value, both yours and other people's. It is the conviction that life is worth living—and worth living well. Individuals with a low sense of significance feel that their existence is irrelevant and that if they did not exist, it would make little difference in the world. Feelings of insignificance are predictors of depression, loneliness, and suicidal ideation.[20] Those who have a strong sense of significance feel important, not in comparison to other people, but in terms of their value and capacity to make positive contributions to the world around them.

Purpose is a sense that your life has direction, that you have an overarching aim or set of aims that you are striving toward. A sense of purpose is something like having a theme or themes to your life that become actionable through the goals you strive for and toward which you direct your best time and effort. Princeton philosopher Susan Wolf describes purpose as arising "from active engagement in projects of worth, which links us to our world in a positive way."[21]

Certitude is the sense that your existence and your life make sense. It is the belief that your life is predictable and consistent enough that you understand the vital associations and connections among important events, experiences, and interactions. Certitude provides a sense that even in the face of uncertainties and chaos, there is a meaningful order and intelligibility underlying your life.

Spirituality is the belief that there is a numinous, divine, or transcendent dimension to existence.[22] Spirituality, as social scientists define it, is the ways people search for and connect with the Sacred, the Divine, God, Ultimate Truth, or another understanding of a higher power, force, or essence.[23] In its best expressions, spirituality guides people toward higher, better, fuller ways of living and being in the world. Religious faith is, of course, one pathway to spirituality.

Dedicated practices (chapter eight) and engaged practices (chapter nine) focus on how you can strengthen your sense of purpose, significance, and certitude through simple, everyday activities. Joyful practices (chapter ten) are wise ways to bring spirituality into the rhythm of your daily life.

Moving Forward on Your Wellbeing Journey

This is a good time to either take the short wellbeing assessment I have included on page 49 or practice Map Your Days. Both will help you step back and consider where there are opportunities for you to strengthen your wellbeing.

If you take the assessment, an area with a score of 4 or lower is a dimension of your wellbeing that needs to be restored or improved. A score between 5 and 7 indicates a dimension of your wellbeing you can grow or take to new levels. A score of 8 or higher indicates you have high wellbeing on that dimension.

After you have identified where you're going, read the chapter about the practices that can help you step easy on that journey. The image that follows, which maps each category of wise practice onto the dimension of wellbeing it can improve and strengthen, will help you find the right chapter or chapters.

Read the appropriate chapter or chapters once. This will help you understand how those practices can help you meet your wellbeing need or goal. Then, read the chapter again and focus on selecting a practice, maybe a couple, that sounds like it is wise for you. And then, step easy. Get in your steps as often as you can, ideally each day. Do the practice regularly for at least a couple of weeks. Get into a rhythm and allow the practice to find a place in your daily life. From there, keep stepping easy so the benefits build up.

Keep in mind that practice, not perfection, is what works. Step back once every month or two to appreciate how you have grown and how your wellbeing has improved. Taking the Lasting Wellbeing Assessment again or practicing Map Your Days would be good ways to capture the improvement you have made, and also help you decide where you want to go next on your journey. Then, come back here to find the wise practices that will help you take those next steps.

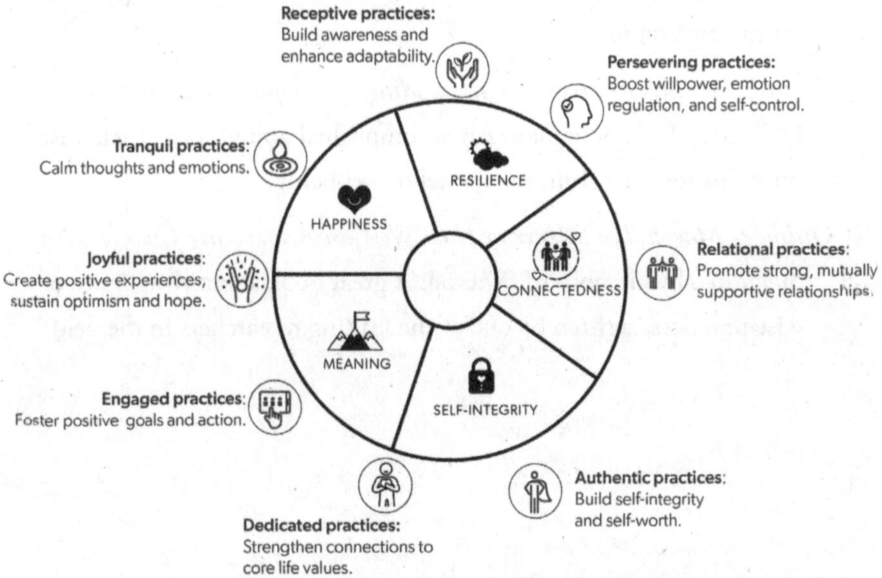
Receptive practices: Build awareness and enhance adaptability.
Persevering practices: Boost willpower, emotion regulation, and self-control.
Tranquil practices: Calm thoughts and emotions.
RESILIENCE
HAPPINESS
Joyful practices: Create positive experiences, sustain optimism and hope.
CONNECTEDNESS
Relational practices: Promote strong, mutually supportive relationships.
MEANING
Engaged practices: Foster positive goals and action.
SELF-INTEGRITY
Authentic practices: Build self-integrity and self-worth.
Dedicated practices: Strengthen connections to core life values.

As you must for all journeys, you have to take a step to begin, so now's the time for you to do so. Trust the practices you choose, trust your journey. Take easy steps for a while, say a month or two, and then step back again. I am confident you will begin to notice the progress you have made on your wellbeing journey.

FURTHER READING

Happiness: Unlocking the Mysteries of Psychological Wealth by Ed Diener and Robert Biswas-Diener: A seminal book written by the world's foremost experts on happiness.

What Contributes to a Life Well-Lived? by the Global Flourishing Study, www.globalflourishingstudy.com/wp-content/uploads/2025/04/GFS_Report.pdf: A comprehensive study of wellbeing across twenty-two nations.

Flourish: A Visionary New Understanding of Happiness and Well-Being by Martin E. P. Seligman: An accomplished and visionary scientist offers his forward-thinking model of wellbeing.

Ordinary Magic: The Science of How We Can Achieve Big Change with Small Acts by Gregory M. Walton: A great book about the science of wise practices, written by one of the leading researchers in the field.

The Lasting Wellbeing Assessment

The following assessment, based on the original 350-question assessment I used in my research, is a good way to step back, see where you are on your wellbeing journey, and identify where you might want to journey next. Researchers want to be extremely precise in their measurements, and that takes a lot of questions. For our purposes here, however, answering 350 questions isn't necessary. Based on statistical analysis, these ten core questions will provide you with a good estimate of your wellbeing.

How to Take the Assessment: There are two questions for each dimension of wellbeing. Select the answer that best represents your wellbeing right now and record the number next to that answer. Then add the numbers from both questions. That's your wellbeing score on that dimension. A score of 4 or lower indicates this is a dimension of your wellbeing that needs to be restored or improved. Focus on these dimensions first. A score of 5 to 7 indicates a dimension of wellbeing you can grow or strengthen. Focus on these dimensions after taking care of any areas of need. Eight and higher means you are doing well, so for the time being, you might focus on other dimensions.

I have listed the wise practice chapters related to each dimension in parentheses.

Happiness *(chapter three, "Tranquil Practices," and chapter ten, "Joyful Practices")*

What are most days like for you?

5—My daily life is awesome!

4—My days are mostly good.

3—Eh, it's a mix, some good and some bad.

2—I'm beginning to feel overwhelmed by daily life.

1—Daily life has left me used up and burned out.

How stressful is life for you right now?

5—Most of the time life is stress free and easy.

4—I face some stressors, but nothing I can't handle.

3—Stress comes and goes, but sometimes it can be a lot.

2—I can feel stress building, and I'm concerned about it.

1—I am often overwhelmed by stress.

Happiness total = ________

Resilience *(chapter four, "Receptive Practices," and chapter five, "Persevering Practices")*

How do you usually feel when life gets difficult?

5—I am always ready for any challenge.

4—I can handle most problems well.

3—Sometimes I'm OK, sometimes I'm not.

2—Worried and uncertain about what to do.

1—Completely overwhelmed.

Imagine you have to fast for a day and someone offered you one of your favorite foods.

5—I wouldn't be tempted at all.

4—It would be hard to fight my impulse, but I could resist.

3—I hope I could resist, but I'm not sure.

2—I would probably give in, then feel bad afterward.

1—I would definitely eat it.

Resilience total = ________

Connectedness *(chapter six, "Relational Practices")*

Do you have people you can really count on?

5—I have many people who really love me.

4—I have several close friends.

3—I have people I could call in an emergency.

2—I'm mostly going through life solo.

1—It's just me against the world.

How would you describe your immediate family?

5—I am part of a very loving, supportive, and caring family.

4—I am very close to some of my family, but not to others.

3—My family and I are cordial, but we don't really know each other.

2—I rarely see my family, and when I do, it can be very tense.

1—I am very disconnected from my family.

Connectedness total = ________

Self-Integrity *(chapter seven, "Authentic Practices," and chapter eight, "Dedicated Practices")*

How do you feel about yourself right now?

5—I feel awesome and super confident.

4—Overall, I think I'm a good person.

3—It depends; sometimes I feel pretty good, but other times I feel the opposite.

2—Kind of shaky—sometimes I struggle with self-worth.

1—I don't feel good about myself at all.

I see myself as

5—Strong and self-confident.

4—Able to stand up for myself in tough situations.

3—Lacking confidence sometimes.

2—Someone who is easily intimidated.

1—Someone who often worries I have done or said something wrong.

Self-Integrity total = ________

Meaning *(chapter eight, "Dedicated Practices"; chapter nine, "Engaged Practices"; and chapter ten, "Joyful Practices")*

How would you describe your sense of purpose in life?

5—I have a clear and strong sense of purpose that I am living each day.

4—Most days, I am able to do things that are important to me.

3—I am searching for a purpose I can really commit to.

2—Most of my daily activities are unimportant and meaningless.

1—I'm lost and wandering aimlessly through life.

How would you describe your core values?

5—I have a clearly defined set of core values that guide my everyday life.

4—I have a strong sense of what matters most to me.

3—I have some idea of what I believe in, but I'm not sure.

2—I have no idea what I really believe in.

1—I think life is meaningless and nothing really matters.

Meaning total = ________

CHAPTER THREE

Tranquil Practices

Dealing Well with Acute Stress

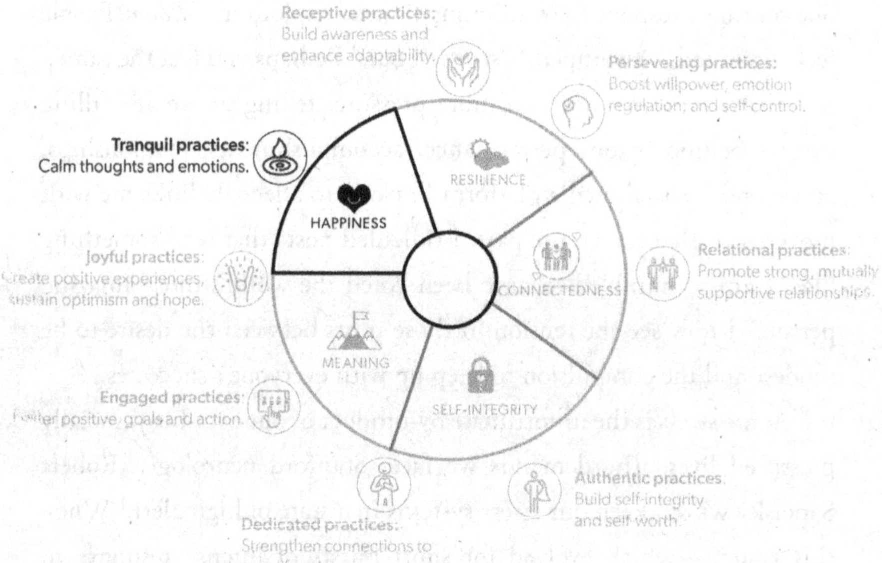

For many of us, the rapid pace of work and life creates heavy demands to make quick decisions, juggle priorities, and go-go-go. Multitasking is essential to making it through the day. Emails, texts, and phone calls contend for our attention. Technology stretches our days so that even when we are "off the clock," work lurks in the back of our minds. To-do lists lengthen, and we lack the time and energy to get everything done.

I see this in the hallways of my university, which often seem more like hospital emergency departments. While I have never heard of an educational emergency—"Professor Bloom, we need you to teach, STAT!"—people rush by with strained expressions as if they are responding to some kind of campus code blue. When I ask, "How are you?" people usually blurt out something like "I am so busy!" Recently, one colleague responded by miming his head exploding—*Boom!* People feel "slammed," "swamped," "stressed out." Perhaps you feel the same.

Social pressures heap on more pressure, telling us we are falling further behind in our performance, accomplishments, relationships, and more. A social media platform I belong to allegedly links me with movers and shakers. In the past, I ridiculed posts that read something like "I am so humbled to have been voted the world's most amazing person." I now see the tension in those posts between the desire to be modest and the compulsion to keep up with everyone's successes.

Acute stress is the unfortunate by-product of our over-busy, socially pressured lives. The demands we face, Stanford neurologist Robert Sapolsky writes, keep our stress systems in a state of high alert.[1] When this system—which evolved for short bursts of intense response to life-threatening dangers—never shuts off, it erodes our wellbeing. We don't sleep well, leaving us chronically exhausted. We can't focus on simple tasks like writing an email or reading a book. We worry more, agonizing over the past and fretting about the future. We overreact and turn everyday events like long checkout lines or traffic jams into major ordeals. We feel edgy and brittle; everything irritates, frustrates, or worries us. Over long periods, stress accumulates and becomes a chronic part of our wellbeing journey. Chronic stress (the focus of chapters four and five) can crescendo into panic attacks, anxiety, or burnout. With tranquil practices, we can defuse acute stress and keep it from building up.

Several years ago, I overextended myself and nearly burned out. I had committed to too many projects. I was working sixteen-hour days, even on the weekends. I went to bed overwhelmed and exhausted and woke up several times throughout the night with my mind churning. I knew my chronic exhaustion and severely diminished work capacities were two symptoms of burnout. On the verge of the third symptom—despondency and despair—I kept up the grind but fell further behind each day.

As I rushed out the door one morning, my wife, Kim, stopped me, put her hands on my chest, and said, "You can't keep going, Matt. You have to go hiking. Now!" Backcountry hiking can be deeply restorative for me. Out on the trail, the worries of everyday life fall away. The rhythm of hiking calms my emotions and relaxes my tense body. I sleep soundly outside.

I knew Kim was right. It was summer. I had vacation time. But I started to protest. She pushed me, hard, to get my attention and said, "GO!"

Two days later I was hiking in the Blue Ridge Mountains.

The Massanutten Trail is a remote, rugged, seventy-mile loop. I needed solitude and expected to find it there. The trail wanders over clear streams, through deep mountain passages, and past small caves hidden in the rocky terrain—a great *Lord of the Rings* setting.

Backcountry hiking requires simplifying, so I only carried necessities: water, food, camp stove, extra clothes, hammock, and sleeping bag. I have learned that boiling my life down to the bare minimum, as scholar and hiker Belden Lane writes, creates space to release "the interior baggage I bring along on the trail."[2] I needed to let go of several heavy loads.

I carried two additional items—an anthology of poems and a book of spiritual writings—and stopped several times a day to read and reflect. The poems inspired hope and wonder, and the book prompted me to think deeply about my life.

Days began with a simple breakfast and an hour of reading. I then packed up and set out to hike. I stopped periodically to rest, snack, and read again. At day's end I set up camp, made a simple meal, and watched the sunset through the trees. At dark, I climbed into my hammock and drifted off into restful sleep.

Day five began with a long ascent to a mountain summit. It would take most of the day, so I hiked a bit slower. Early in the afternoon when I was sitting comfortably on a rock, I heard a loud noise. It sounded like an animal crashing through the forest. Suddenly, I saw a man pushing a mountain bike up the steep trail, breathing hard and sweating profusely.

"I didn't expect to see anybody!" he shouted.

"Me neither," I replied, "but I'm ready to hike, so you can take this spot to rest."

He looked at me with bewilderment, then shouted, "No, goddammit! You can never stop pushing! I have to keep pushing!"

And he did. Up the trail, still pushing, breathing hard, sweating, and swearing.

As the quiet resettled around me, I reflected on that brief and perplexing encounter. I realized I was like him. Keep pushing no matter what—no matter the exhaustion, no matter the consequences, no matter whether I cared about the summit. It was a gift of insight to see myself and my life in a new way. When I returned, I shared this story with a close friend. He bought me a small model of a mountain bike as a reminder. It's sitting on my desk now as I write.

It's unusual to be able to get away like that, but you don't need to go to the extremes I did. A simple tranquil practice would have kept me well and can do the same for you. The day I returned home, I began a breath meditation practice. Hiking is still a favorite, as is a poetry reading practice. I make better choices about work now, but life still gets messy, so my daily tranquil practices are essential for my wellbeing journey.

Tranquil practices can foster a peaceful state of mind, calm emotional turmoil, restore your capacity to focus, and turn off your stress system. Even short periods of tranquil practice can yield significant benefits for your brain and, consequently, your body.

How Your Brain Processes Stress

Our brains are incredibly complex organs. They produce thoughts, personalities, identities, dreams, ideas, and much more. Although you may think these amazing capacities are part of your brain's main purpose, they aren't. Your brain's main function is to keep you alive. Thinking is more like a fancy accessory (a really nice one, for sure) than a core component. Your stress system is an essential part of this survival function—that is, when it works well.[3] To understand how your brain and stress system are *supposed* to work, we will use a simple exercise originally created by UCLA research psychiatrist Daniel Siegel, which I have adapted a bit here.

Begin by interlacing the fingers of your two hands as if you were praying or holding hands with yourself. Now, tuck your thumbs between your palms and bring your wrists together. This is a simplified model of your brain and nervous system.

Your wrists represent your spinal cord, which brings information from your five senses (vision, hearing, smell, taste, touch), muscles, and organs into your brain. Everything you "know" about what is going on inside and outside of you travels through your spinal cord or nerves to get into your brain.

The base of your palms represents your brainstem, which is the area responsible for regulating most of your body's vital life functions, including balance, reflexes, blood pressure, sleep, and swallowing. Your brainstem works without your conscious involvement to keep your heart pumping, your lungs breathing, and your digestive system operating. Because your brain's main purpose is to keep you alive, its stem is the first place that sensory information passes through.

Your thumbs symbolize the limbic region of your brain, the next place sensory information goes. This region has several important functions. It is the source of basic drives like hunger, thirst, avoiding pain, and seeking pleasure, which can be powerful motivators.

Your limbic region is the seat of your emotions: happiness, anger, sadness, joy, dejection, excitement, and fear. Beyond the profound experiences that emotions create, they are also, as Yale University research psychologist Marc Brackett describes, "a form of information.

They're like news reports from inside our psyches, sending messages about what's going on inside the unique person that is each of us in response to whatever internal or external events we're experiencing. They motivate us."[4]

Positive emotions like inspiration, interest, and cheerfulness signal that all is well. Positive emotions keep you moving forward and at times can motivate you to go beyond what you normally think is possible. They can move you deeply and are essential to life's most meaningful experiences. Negative emotions signal something is wrong and motivate you to take corrective action. Fear, for example, impels us to seek safety, and anger drives us to confront its source. We respond to negative emotions more strongly and remember them more clearly, and their effects last longer. This is why conditions like depression and PTSD can be difficult to overcome—they are powered by negative emotions.

The limbic region is also your brain's watchdog. University of California at San Francisco stress researcher Elissa Epel writes that our brains "are wired . . . to look for danger, to be vigilant, because the world—whether ancient jungles or modern cities—has always been full of uncertainty and danger."[5] The limbic region does this by constantly scanning incoming sensory signals for information about your environment. Signs of danger elicit a surge of negative emotions that launches your stress system and activates its emergency (*fight-flight-freeze*) response. Your body gets ready to react to the threat—your heart rate and blood pressure increase dramatically, your pain response shuts down, energy pours into your muscles, and your brain narrows its focus to the threat and nothing more. Once the danger abates, your limbic region shuts down the stress system.

The problem we face, as Sapolsky describes, is that the pressures of modern life can cause our stress systems to remain activated "for months on end, worrying about mortgages, relationships, and promotions." When this happens, "the stress-response can become more damaging than the stressor itself."[6] This "always on" condition creates what I call the limbic loop. Worrying unleashes negative emotions that activate your stress system and emergency response, thrusting your body into crisis mode. Your thoughts lock on to potential threats, your worrying increases, negative emotions continue to surge, and the limbic loop turns faster. Left unaddressed, the limbic loop can create mental health challenges such as chronic stress syndrome, persistent anxiety, and burnout.

Let's move now to your interlaced fingers, which represent the two halves of your cerebrum, the biggest and smartest part of your brain. Conscious thoughts form here, including creative ideas, rational decisions, intelligent conclusions, detailed plans, snap judgments, deep insights, and imaginative forethoughts. Your understanding of yourself, other people, and the world around you is also formed here.

Sometimes your cerebrum wanders off onto thoughts that are distant from what is going on in front of you. Some mind wandering is innocuous, like when you are daydreaming. But mind wandering can also be intense and unpleasant, particularly if it turns into persistent worrying or obsessive thinking. When this happens, your capacity to engage in careful, logical thinking is greatly diminished. Your emotions get drafted into the growing tumult, and you become more distressed. These emotions, in turn, power up your stress system. You are back in the limbic loop. Remarkably, this means that you can activate your emergency response with just your thoughts, when you are sitting safely at your desk or lying quietly in bed, with no real threat lurking.

Look again at your hands. Although there are different parts—wrists, palms, fingers, thumbs—they are interconnected and work together as a coordinated unit. Your brain works in a similarly coordinated way, each region playing its proper role. This is especially true while responding to stressors. When a car swerves into your lane or you accidentally touch a hot stove, you need the lightning-quick reactions of your brainstem and limbic region. But most of the stressors of modern life—an overbearing boss, looming deadlines, financial challenges—require the careful thinking of your cerebrum. With these stressors, you need to intercept any emergency response so you can think about what you should do.

How Tranquil Practices Work

Tranquil practices build your capacity to regulate limbic responses, calm jittery thinking, and ease emotional tension. They refresh your capacity to focus, strengthen your ability to think clearly, and restore your stress system to its proper operating capacity. And they can do all of this with just a few minutes of daily practice.[7]

An experience I had when I first read Sapolsky's *Why Zebras Don't Get Ulcers* illustrates the benefits of tranquil practices. I took his book on a long flight to Southeast Asia to continue my wellbeing research with humanitarian workers. I planned on spending time with a team assigned to areas devastated by natural disasters like typhoons and tsunamis. Teams like this one live and work in traumatized communities to support the difficult process of recovery. They face extremely difficult living and working conditions that pose significant risks for their physical and mental health. The goal of my visit was to learn how to help sustain the wellbeing of these teams.

Renee headed the team I studied. Easygoing, kind, funny, smart, and exceptionally competent, she was a skillful leader who also served on her organization's staff care team. These dual roles made her an ideal partner for my work. In my second week, we took a six-hour trip to a remote village (120 miles over mountainous roads), which gave us time to talk about the wellbeing challenges she and her team experienced. As she described their everyday stressors—shortages of food and water, risk of significant injury from damaged structures, exposure to disease from a variety of pathogens—I thought about Sapolsky's book. Renee and her team faced serious threats, but the team was remarkably calm and upbeat. Even after several weeks on site, the team remained composed and highly effective in their work.

Renee and I talked about how they managed stress. Being a close, highly skilled unit helped tremendously, but she also emphasized the importance of their daily tranquil practice. "Before we head out for work, we start each day meditating," Renee explained. "We gather together and sit in a circle facing each other. Each day one of us volunteers to read a quote, poem, or Scripture to ground and inspire us, and that person leads the meditation. We start by focusing on our breathing for ten minutes or so, longer if we have time. Then the leader shares the reading, and we meditate on that for a while. Some days we only have twenty minutes, but most days we can go longer. We end by hugging each other and then we jump into the day feeling peaceful and grounded."

The practice was simple enough that they could do it almost anywhere: in a tent, on an airplane, sitting under a tree. When I asked other team members about it, they agreed that the practice helped them manage stress that would otherwise be overwhelming. Over the time I spent with them, I noticed how team members brought this tranquil practice into their busy days. They would pause for a few minutes to close their eyes and breathe slowly to ground themselves and reconnect with a sense of peace.

Let's explore how you can experience similar benefits from tranquil practices. As you read, keep in mind the two principles of a wise practice, described in chapter one: It should be evidence-based (valid); and it should fit your beliefs, preferences, and lifestyle (personalized). To help you personalize your choice, you will find descriptions of seven different types of tranquil practices throughout this chapter. Empowered with this knowledge, you will be able to find at least one that will work for you.

One of the most common tranquil practices is breath-focused meditation, which can be done in as little as five minutes. As you feel ready, practice for longer periods. You may also adapt this practice the way Renee's team did by including a segment in which you focus on a special reading.

BREATH-FOCUSED MEDITATION

Begin by getting into a relaxed, comfortable position, either seated or lying down. Let your hands rest in a gentle position and allow your breath to flow normally. After a few breaths, notice the rhythm of your breathing. Continue in this relaxed, natural way for a few moments. If you find yourself thinking about something else, simply focus again on your breath.

When you feel ready, follow the passing of air as you inhale and exhale, noticing how your breath feels as it moves in and out of your nose. Keep breathing naturally as you focus on air moving into your body. You can gently move your attention from your nose to the way your shoulders, chest, and abdomen move as you breathe. Again here, focus on the way breathing feels in these different places. Anytime your mind wanders, gently bring your focus back to your breath. When you are ready to finish, take a final breath or two, then slowly open your eyes and reorient yourself to the space you are in.

A study of multitaskers shows how even short experiences with tranquil practices can be helpful.[8] Thomas Gorman and Shawn Green, psychologists at the University of Wisconsin, recruited 1,600 students who were heavy multitaskers (defined as engaging in it every day) and who had never meditated. They used a battery of tests to measure the students' mind wandering. Then, half the students were told to browse the web for ten minutes, and the other half were taught a simple breath meditation practice. They counted their breaths from one to nine and repeated this sequence for ten minutes. After browsing or practicing breath meditation, the students were assessed again. The web browsers recorded either no change or an increase in mind wandering, but the tranquil breathers showed a nearly 50 percent reduction—after their first time with a tranquil practice and only ten minutes!

Box breathing is another breath-based practice that is as simple and effective as the practice used in Gorman and Green's study.

BOX BREATHING

Begin by finding a comfortable position—sitting, lying down, even standing can work. Breathe out slowly through pursed lips, releasing all the air from your lungs. Then, breathe in slowly through your nose as you count to four in your head. Notice how the air fills your lungs and stomach. This builds the first side of the box. The second side of the box is created by holding your breath for a count of four. Build the third side by exhaling for another count of four. Create the fourth side of the box by holding your breath again for a count of four. Build several boxes. To help you stay focused, as you build each side, you can draw it on the palm of one hand using the first finger of the other hand.

Tranquil practices work through two main neuropsychological channels or pathways: by fostering present-moment attention and by developing the capacity for meta-awareness.[9] Fostering present-moment attention is the best pathway for most people and the one we will discuss first.

Present-Moment Attention

Practices that work through this neuropsychological channel include mindfulness meditation, yoga, relaxation techniques, and breath meditation. When you practice present-moment attention, you are using your powerful cerebrum to keep your attention and focus on the here and now, thinking less about the past or future.[10] A mindful eating practice created by Jon Kabat-Zinn, a psychologist and pioneering stress researcher at the University of Massachusetts Chan Medical School, was designed to introduce people to practicing present-moment attention. If you are new to tranquil practices, it can be a great way to get a sense of what they are like.

EATING MINDFULLY

To begin, you will need three small pieces of food like raisins, nuts, or bits of dry cereal. Start by observing the pieces of food. Take a close look, noticing the color, texture, and feel of each piece and the aromas arising from them. Spend a few minutes looking at each, noticing similarities and differences. Also notice what you are thinking and feeling. Goofy? Calm? Uncomfortable? Excited? Name the thoughts and emotions as if you are tagging them. If you catch your mind wandering, acknowledge those thoughts and return your attention to the food.

When you feel ready, take one piece and hold it up to eat. Observe how your body responds as you anticipate eating it, then slowly eat the first piece, savoring the taste and texture. Pause for a moment when you feel the impulse to swallow and examine how that feels. After eating that first piece, sense how your body is one piece of food heavier. Slowly eat the second, taking time and care to savor its taste and texture, and attend to how it is both the same as and different from the first piece. After swallowing, sense how your body has changed. Repeat with the third piece. End by taking a few moments to reflect on the experience.

Building the capacity for present-moment attention helps restore your stress system to its proper working order. During a tranquil practice, your limbic region is less active and reactive. Your emergency response switches to standby mode and turns off your hair-trigger reactions, which makes room for calmer, cooler, and more collected responding.

Neuroscience research indicates that regular tranquil practices also strengthen the integrative functioning that is essential for the brain to operate optimally.[11] This includes strengthening the connections between the limbic region and cerebrum. Your stress system is still operative, but it will launch only when real danger is present. You have a heightened ability for controlled, thoughtful responses to life's stressors. In other words, making a tranquil practice a regular part of your wellbeing journey keeps your stress system in top working condition.

Body scanning exercises are especially helpful for calming your stress response and can be a great place to start cultivating present-moment attention. I sometimes use these while sitting on an airplane, and they can work wonders after a challenging day or on a bumpy flight.

BODY SCANNING

Get into a comfortable position sitting, lying down, standing—whatever feels best. Close your eyes and allow your body to relax. You might imagine your body sinking into the bed or couch or feel your body resting safely on the chair. Take three or four deep breaths and allow your body to relax and rest a bit more. Begin the body scan by focusing on your feet. Feel the pressure of your feet on the bed or couch or floor. Notice how your feet and toes feel—any sensations of pressure, vibration, weight, temperature, and tension in your muscles. Then, relax your toes and feet fully, imagining the muscles slowly easing as tension flows away. After a few moments, move your attention to your ankles and notice the sensations there. Take your time. When you are ready, allow your ankles to fully relax. After a few moments, move your attention to your lower legs and take a few moments to repeat the process of observing the sensations you feel there. Relax the muscles there, perhaps again imagining the tension flowing out of your lower legs. Repeat this observation and relaxation process as you slowly scan the other major areas of your body: upper legs, hips, abdomen, chest, neck, shoulders, arms, hands—all the way to face and head. Pause to notice the sensations in each part of your body, relaxing the muscles in each area. Allow your entire body to sink deeply into the place you are lying or sitting. Finish by opening your eyes and becoming aware of the space around you.

Present-moment attention also strengthens your capacity to regulate your emotions, which is essential for managing stress well. We can experience hundreds of different emotions. For example, being afraid, scared, startled, terrified, petrified, frightened, alarmed, apprehensive, uneasy, perturbed, nervous, jittery, and shaky are each different emotions, as are anger, rage, fury, wrath, indignation, vexation, umbrage, annoyance, irritability, frustration, and exasperation. Each of these emotions is a different experience and has its own proper response. The best way to respond to terror is different from dealing well with apprehension or unease. Responding well when you are furious is different from handling irritation appropriately.

Ask someone stuck in the limbic loop what they are feeling, and they will use broad terms like "stressed," "burned out," or "bad." Feeling "bad" leaves you to deal with a large and amorphous experience; you cannot adequately identify what feeling "bad" means or what caused it, so all you can do is try to deny, ignore, or repress your emotions. Unfortunately, this fuels bad feelings and keeps your stress system on high alert. Being more emotionally granular makes you more adept at understanding and controlling your emotions. Assigning appropriate and specific labels to your emotions communicates more clearly to your brain your perception of a situation. This stops the full-throttle flow of negative emotions and allows you to mentally detach from the situation.

You are also less likely to feel overwhelmed in challenging or stressful situations because identifying and accepting negative emotions disarms them. Neuroscience research shows that emotional granularity can calm the emotion center of your limbic region (your amygdala), making it less reactive and less noisy. By turning down negative emotions, you shut off the energy supply to the limbic loop.

Practicing present-moment attention also strengthens your capacity to regulate your thoughts. During tranquil practices, your cerebrum is both active and calm. You think with clarity and composure, which increases your capacity to control your thoughts and mind wandering. Over time, you'll learn to keep your mind from wandering because you decide where to direct your attention. This, in turn, empowers you to engage in more flexible and effective responses to stressful situations. You can step back to gain perspective on what is happening, think carefully and clearly about options for responding, and maintain the ability to pivot to a different approach as needed. Instead of fleeing, freezing, fighting, or acting in some other impulsive way, you can respond thoughtfully and effectively.

Some people, including me, find it easier to control our focus when we are moving compared to when we are sitting or lying still. Hiking is one of my favorite tranquil practices because I can focus on the movement of my legs, which muscles are being used, where I am tense or relaxed, and how the swinging of my arms feels. Other practices like yoga, dancing, and tai chi can also be adapted as movement-based tranquil practices that create present-moment attention. Walking meditation is among the most common movement-based tranquil practices, and it is very flexible because it can be done inside or outside. I have done it in a hotel room, in the aisle of an airplane on long flights, and on those good days out on the hiking trail. A simple walking practice is a good place to begin if you find it easier to focus when you are moving.

WALKING MEDITATION

Find a place that allows you to walk in a small circle or back and forth in a short line. It should be relatively peaceful so you won't be disturbed (or observed if you want to practice in private). Begin simply by walking gently and slowly, paying attention to each foot as it lands softly on the ground. Place your arms in a comfortable position, such as clasping hands behind you. The core of walking meditation is to think deliberately about the things you normally do automatically when walking. At first this might feel awkward, even ridiculous, but the goal is to focus deeply.

Each step has four basic components, and in walking meditation, you move slowly through each one: lifting one foot off the ground, moving that foot forward slowly, placing the foot deliberately but softly on the ground, and shifting your body weight onto that foot. As you go through this process, try to focus your attention on the sensations that you normally would not notice, like the movement of muscles, how your body responds to each movement, and your breath as it moves in and out of your lungs. Repeat this slow, focused process step-by-step. You might begin with four steps, then in successive practices add more.

Visualization or guided-imagery practices are also wise ways to calm your thoughts and focus your attention on the present moment. These involve imagining yourself in a beautiful, peaceful, or sacred place. The goal is to build a rich mental image of the place, including all the positive sensations—feelings, smells, sounds, sights, tastes—that you would experience if you were there in person. They work because your brain treats what it "sees" in your imagination as if it were happening in real time. I use these kinds of practices when I am having trouble sleeping. I visualize myself scuba diving over a beautiful coral reef. I feel the warm water supporting me, and I take the same kind of calm breaths I use when I am actually scuba diving. At some point, I fall asleep as I enjoy my imaginary underwater world.

VISUALIZATION

Begin by getting into a comfortable position, sitting, lying down, whatever feels best to you. Then, close your eyes and take a few slow, deep breaths. Visualize yourself lying on a white sandy beach. It's a beautiful day. Imagine the wonderful aspects of that experience: the warm sun, the soft sand, the gentle breeze. Relax and listen for a while. Perhaps you hear waves gently coming to shore—allow yourself to experience those peaceful sounds. You might see and hear birds and experience their brilliant colors and lovely songs. Take a deep breath and notice the fragrances that are present. Imagine the beautiful turquoise water. Perhaps you go out into the water and feel its gentle warmth. Spend time in this lovely place and allow yourself to indulge in a vivid daydream of what being at the beach would feel like.

You can visualize any place that you find beautiful and peaceful; it doesn't have to be a beach. A quiet meadow, beautiful mountain vista, or lovely flower garden will work just as well.

There is one more tranquil practice, loving-kindness meditation, that has received significant research support. It can also be highly effective in cultivating compassion and goodwill for yourself and others.

LOVING-KINDNESS MEDITATION

Begin by sitting or lying in a relaxed posture and taking several deep breaths. After a few moments, bring your attention to the center of your chest, where your heart is. You might place a hand gently there. As you do this, silently offer thoughts of love and kindness to yourself. Slowly repeat phrases like, "May I be safe. May I be happy. May I be healthy. May I be joyful. May I be loving." Choose phrases and words that feel right for you and that are easy to remember. Form thoughts and intentions that convey love, warmth, compassion, and care to yourself. You might imagine feelings of warmth that move from your chest into the other areas of your body, all the way to your toes and head.

Continue this practice by shifting your attention to someone you care about deeply. Offer those same phrases, "May [name of person] be safe . . . happy . . . healthy . . . joyful . . . loving." As you do this, you can imagine that you are sitting next to or holding them, or perhaps you might imagine waves of warmth and love flowing toward that person. Include as many people as you wish, focusing on one at a time and offering the same phrases. End by turning your attention to sending compassion to all people, "May all people be safe . . . happy . . . etc." End with a few moments of quiet and perhaps an expression of gratitude for the practice.

Over time, you can try to send love to a person with whom you have some difficulty. I have found that adding challenging people into my practice changes my attitude toward them for the better.

Meta-Awareness

A second neuropsychological pathway through which tranquil practices work emerges when you strengthen your ability to engage in *meta-awareness*.[12] This is a more advanced pathway, usually requiring training from an experienced teacher, so I will introduce it only briefly here.

Meta-awareness is the capacity to shut down judgments, evaluations, inner critiques, and other negative thought patterns. It entails mentally stepping away from your thoughts and emotions, as if you were observing them from a distance, so that you can see and think about them in a detached, dispassionate way.

In most situations, we are aware of what we are thinking about but remain unaware of the mental processes we are using to do it. Here's an example: Consider what happens when you watch a captivating movie at home. You can become so swept away by the action on the screen that you lose awareness of where you are and what is going on around you. That is normal awareness—the movie has your full attention. Now, imagine watching that same movie while also maintaining awareness of being in your home, sitting on a particular chair or sofa. You are aware of the specific feelings and thoughts you are experiencing as you watch. You are enjoying the movie but still remaining aware of what is going on around you. That is meta-awareness.

While it can be great to get swept up in a movie, it is another thing to get swept up by worries, fears, and other negative mental states. Meta-awareness builds your capacity for nonreactive, nonjudgmental thinking. The motto "Don't believe everything you think" is often used to describe the goal of practicing meta-awareness. Over time, you learn how to acknowledge worries, fears, and anxieties without being swept up by them. In this way, you can deal with them productively.

With regular practice, meta-awareness leads to what researchers call "the brain on silent," a mental stillness in which thinking is reduced to a minimum.[13] This creates the capacity to respond in an even-minded and even-tempered way to stressors. Consider the example of driving in heavy traffic, when suddenly another car cuts in front of you. The most common response is yelling at the aggressive driver and laying on the car horn. In this response, you drive with the limbic loop throttled up, fueled by anger and perhaps a desire for revenge. By building the capacity for meta-awareness, you would take appropriate evasive action, like slowing down or braking to avoid a collision, while noting the actions of the other driver without judgment or anger. Your drive remains safe, and you remain calm.

A research study of master meditator Matthieu Ricard showcased this capacity. A famous Buddhist monk, Ricard is known as "the happiest man in the world," an ironic title given Buddhism's emphasis on detaching from worldly experiences. More germane to his religious beliefs are his more than forty years of daily Buddhist meditation practice. In the study, Ricard entered an hourlong meditative state that he described as "very vast, clear, vivid and lucid, and fully resting in the moment."[14] In other words, he was in a state of full meta-awareness. At a randomly selected time, a "startle stimulus," a sudden, gunshot-like sound, came through loudspeakers located behind his head. The sound was sufficiently loud to produce a strong defensive reaction in most people. A camera recorded Ricard's facial expressions, and electrodes measured his heart rate, blood flow, and muscle and skin responses. This experiment was repeated several times, and the results were the same. Remarkably, Ricard never showed a startle response. He remained peaceful and calm: no muscle twitch, no change in heart rate, nothing but a soft smile on his face.

Practices that foster meta-awareness include insight or Vipassana meditation, Zen zazen, and Vajrayana visualization. It is worth trying a meta-awareness practice if you find yourself drawn to them, but they are best undertaken with the guidance of a skilled teacher.

A Note on Religious and Spiritual Practices

Most religious traditions have spiritual practices that engage one or both of the tranquil pathways. Some of the mindfulness meditation practices that are popular today, like breath-focused meditation, have their roots in Buddhism. As I have described, these secular versions can be very helpful for managing stress, but other benefits arise when they are practiced in keeping with their original religious purposes. If you are religiously observant, you might find the spiritual practices of your tradition especially helpful.

Examples in the Christian tradition are centering and contemplative prayer; *lectio divina*, the slow, imaginative reading of sacred texts; and prayer labyrinths, a form of walking meditation. Muslim practices include *taffakur*, pondering on Allah's love and compassion; and *murāqabah*, opening one's heart to receive divine truths, spiritual enlightenment, or other spiritual gifts. Other traditions, including Judaism, Hinduism, Baha'i, Jainism, and Taoism, have spiritual practices that can be very helpful for their adherents.

Some Cautions About Tranquil Practices

The hype around mindfulness meditation too often portrays it as a wonder practice, a cure-all for everything. But researchers are adamant that tranquil practices are not a panacea for every kind of wellbeing need. Furthermore, while tranquil practices will work well for most of us, they are not appropriate for all of us. In some cases, people have bad experiences with a particular tranquil practice, including uncomfortable thoughts and feelings, increased worry and anxiety, and in a few cases, more serious psychological problems. You should stop any tranquil practice that causes uncomfortable experiences. This is why it is so important to find one that is wise for you.

Also, please remember that none of the practices in this book are a replacement for qualified mental healthcare. If you have any concerns about whether a tranquil practice is appropriate for you, or if you are experiencing a serious mental health challenge, please seek the assistance of a trained professional.

KEY INSIGHTS

Our hardwired capacity to respond to acute stress is the *fight-flight-freeze* system. Its normal operation is to become highly activated when danger is present, and then shut down quickly as soon as the danger has passed. Modern life, however, often pushes us into a constant state of emergency, so our stress response is always in high gear.

The main pathway through which tranquil practices work is fostering present-moment attention. This is the capacity to calm your thoughts and emotions, and mentally detach from the stressful experience.

Practices like breath meditation and loving kindness are great places to start. They can be done when you are stopped at a red light, on the train or subway, or during any other natural pause in your daily life.

FURTHER READING

The Stress Prescription: Seven Days to More Joy and Ease by Elissa Epel: An engaging exploration of stress and what to do about it.

Altered Traits: Science Reveals How Meditation Changes Your Mind, Brain, and Body by Daniel Goleman and Richard J. Davidson: A science-based guide to mindfulness meditation.

Full Catastrophe Living: Using the Wisdom of Your Body and Mind to Face Stress, Pain, and Illness by Jon Kabat-Zinn: The seminal scientific exploration of tranquil practices.

Breath: The New Science of a Lost Art by James Nestor: A good survey of different breath-based tranquil practices.

Aware: The Science and Practice of Presence, the Groundbreaking Meditation Practice by Daniel J. Siegel: A unique but comprehensive approach to developing a tranquil practice.

CHAPTER FOUR

Receptive Practices

Becoming Psychologically Flexible

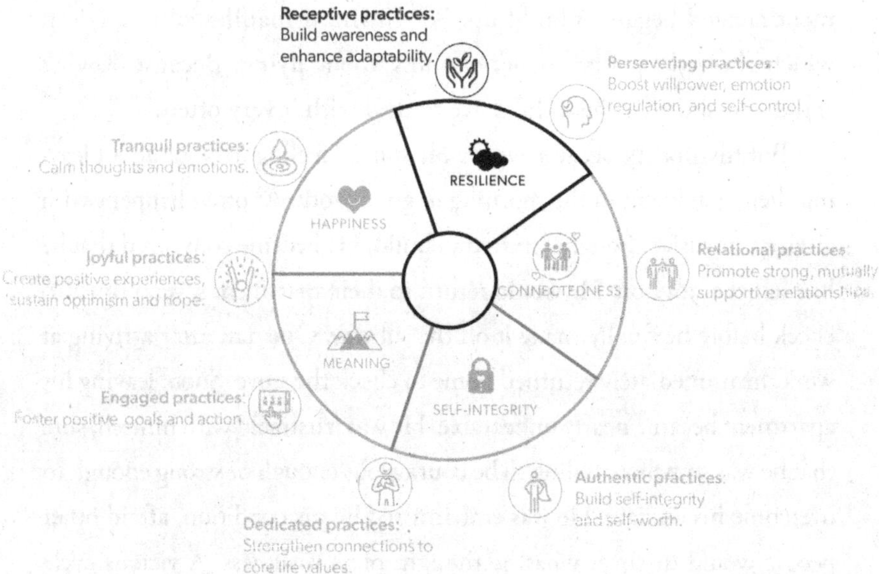

Kevin was a very successful young attorney in Boston. He worked for a prestigious firm, made a nice salary, and lived in the trendy part of the city. His girlfriend was a doctor who would soon finish her residency and join a clinic as an attending physician. They planned to get married the following year. They were popular with their friends. They went to the symphony, ate at chic restaurants, and flew to exotic locations overseas on their vacations. Life seemed to be very good for them, except for Kevin's anxiety, which was getting worse.

Kevin had always been a very conscientious, hardworking student, and he brought that attitude to his work. His boss was a demanding and capricious person, delighted one day with how the cases were going, apoplectic about some "catastrophe" the next. Each day was a terrible experience, and the chronic stress this chaotic work environment created began to build up. For Kevin, it manifested as anxiety, which showed up first as nervousness about flying. Because Kevin's travel was sporadic, he didn't have to deal with it very often.

But his anxiety became worse. He started feeling nervous about leaving their apartment in the morning to go to work. As often happens with anxiety, intrusive thoughts started to build. He became convinced that he had left the stove on. He would return to their apartment several times to check before he finally made it on the subway. One day, after arriving at work, he immediately returned home to check the stove. Soon, leaving his apartment became nearly unbearable. He was frustrated with himself, sure that he was somehow failing to be courageous enough or strong enough to overcome his anxiety. He was embarrassed by his condition, afraid other people would discover what he thought of as weakness. A vicious cycle had begun and Kevin felt he could not extract himself from it. To escape, he needed to develop the capacity for psychological flexibility.

Chronic stress is a prolonged state of distress that diminishes well-being and, over time, impairs mental health. Days are full of difficulties: Problems seem unresolvable, relationships become fraught with conflict, to-do lists grow longer and more complicated. Chronic stress saps resilience and makes us more susceptible to even modest stressors. At its core, chronic stress manifests a chain of negative thoughts and emotions that are experienced as relatively uncontrollable. University of Michigan psychologist Ethan Kross calls this mental chatter, "cyclical negative thoughts and emotions that turn our singular capacity for introspection into a curse rather than a blessing . . . We think about that screwup at work or misunderstanding with a loved one and end up flooded by how bad we feel. Then we think about it again. And again."[1]

Sometimes chronic stress is caused by emotionally troubling experiences from the past. While traumas can begin with an acute stressor, like being in a car accident or physically attacked, it is the chronic stress resulting from those experiences that creates long-term suffering. As Boston University psychiatrist and trauma expert Bessel van der Kolk writes, a distressing experience

> produces actual physiological changes, including a recalibration of the brain's alarm system, an increase in stress hormone activity, and alterations in the system that filters relevant information from irrelevant. We now know that trauma compromises the brain area that communicates the physical, embodied feeling of being alive. These changes explain why traumatized individuals become hyper-vigilant to threat at the expense of spontaneously engaging in their day-to-day lives.[2]

Last, chronic stress can also be created by looming worries and anticipated difficulties such as an upcoming cancer screening, a big deadline at work, or another year-end scramble to finish all of your projects on time. The American Institute of Stress estimates the cost of work-related stress to the American economy at more than $300 billion annually.[3] The American Psychological Association's annual Stress in America survey indicates that 77 percent of American adults report high levels of stress due largely to worries about political turmoil and social divisiveness.[4] A 2023 survey of over six thousand college students reports that 63 percent felt overwhelmed by anxiety during the previous year.[5] Chronic stress can create a host of wellbeing challenges, including anxiety, fatigue, poor sleep quality, poor work performance, and burnout.[6]

Receptive practices help you deal effectively with troubling experiences and increase resilience by increasing your capacity for psychological flexibility. Such flexibility changes the way you interpret and interact with unwanted situations so that you can experience them better. These practices work by increasing your capacity to be aware of troubling thoughts and feelings. They also strengthen your ability to understand the nature of troubling experiences and why you are reacting to them in a particular way, while enhancing your ability to reinterpret difficult life situations in more beneficial ways.

Virtually all situations, from the very best to the very worst, are open to interpretation. We make subjective judgments about what is happening and how it is affecting us and other people. Here's an example of how two people can see the same situation in remarkably different ways. On my way to work one day, I heard on the radio that one of my colleagues, Carl, had won a fully loaded, top-of-the-line SUV, thanks to a local dealership contest. I was thrilled for Carl! How great to win a brand-new luxury vehicle! When I got to work, I immediately went to his office, excited to congratulate him. His door was open, and when I stepped in I could see Carl was clearly in distress. His face was red and he was storming back and forth muttering something. I said, "Congratulations on the new SUV, Carl!"

He looked at me with indignation and almost yelled, "Congratulations? I have to pay [expletive!] gift taxes on the [expletive!] car!"

I told him I would pay the taxes if he would gift me the SUV. He was not amused.

If we see troubling situations the way Carl saw winning a new car, it's unlikely things will get better. We need to see them as Kevin learned to. He was able to escape from the prison of anxiety by using receptive practices that helped him perceive and acknowledge his negative thoughts and emotions. Receptive practices then helped him examine the maladaptive thought patterns that caused those emotions so he could see a path out of his distress. Last, he used persevering practices—the focus of the next chapter—which helped him find more adaptive ways of coping with his worries.

Building Psychological Flexibility

Psychological flexibility is one of the elements of resilience (adaptive coping, the subject of chapter five, is the other). Over time, as your psychological flexibility builds, you will be able to anticipate how adversities might affect you so you can plan positive responses.

Increasing psychological flexibility begins with revisiting your responses after a troubling event has ended by doing a postmortem to understand what you were thinking and feeling. I call this "know after" understanding. For example, after you had an angry outburst at someone, you can step back and review what caused you to get so mad and how you expressed your anger.

Then, as your capacity for psychological flexibility grows, you gain the ability to notice your responses as they are unfolding, when the adverse event is still ongoing. Here, you can take action to mitigate negative reactions and maybe even redirect yourself to respond more positively. I call this "know during" understanding. For example, you feel yourself getting angry, so you pause for a moment, gather your thoughts, calm yourself down a bit, and respond by constructively describing your concerns to the other person.

As your capacity for psychological flexibility becomes even stronger, you can anticipate how you might respond before adversity happens, and you can take preventative measures to ensure you will respond well. I call this a "know before" understanding. For example, you need to discuss a serious concern with another person and you know it's a situation in which you might get angry. You step back from your concerns to try to see the situation from that person's perspective and gain empathy for why they may have responded as they did, and your anger dissipates. You enter the conversation with expressions of kindness and respect for the person, and are able to resolve your concerns amicably. When psychological flexibility empowers you to know before, you can use persevering practices (chapter five) to respond well to difficult situations.

The first step in building psychological flexibility and your capacity to know before is radical acceptance.

Radical Acceptance

Our reaction to troubling experiences is often to try to avoid thinking about or dealing with them. We are flooded with negative thoughts and emotions, and we try desperately to get out of that deluge by mentally, and sometimes physically, running away. As psychologists Sally Winston and Martin Seif write, there is "something very strange and frustrating about your unwanted thoughts: the harder you try to not think them, the louder and more insistent they become." They continue:

> Not wanting the thought, worrying about it, or fighting with it stops it from passing quickly. Chances are, you don't want it because you are upset or turned off by the content. But that is just the beginning. Because you worry about it, reject it, and try to push it out of your mind, it pushes back and becomes a recurring thought or image. After a while, it starts to redirect your attention: It starts arriving with a "whoosh," and feels awful, disgusting, or dreaded. It contains an urgent feeling of needing to get rid of it.[7]

We become immersed in a stream of negative internal talk, which, Kross emphasizes, "concentrates our attention narrowly on the source of our emotional distress," thus stealing the brainpower we need to respond effectively. We jam up our brains with, Kross writes, "the task of listening to our pained inner voice," and so we lack the mental bandwidth to do something helpful about our distress.[8]

So, we get stuck in a downward distress spiral. Something bad happens, and our automatic interpretation is, "This is awful, disgusting, dreadful." We try to push the bad thoughts away and avoid dealing with them. Because "whatever we resist, persists," the situation doesn't get better, and our negative interpretations grow worse. When we try to worry ourselves out of the situation, we are only feeding the troubling thoughts, which then makes us feel worse, which then makes us interpret the situation as even more dire than we originally thought, which . . . you get the idea.

Radical acceptance is fully facing the distressing thoughts and emotions you are experiencing.[9] It involves admitting what you are worried about, afraid of, angry over. Radical acceptance is embracing "THIS SUCKS!" or "I am so sad" or "I am totally pissed off" or whatever you need to say to yourself about what it is like for you to be experiencing the bad, difficult, troublesome, distressing situation. Yes, you can even wallow in your misery for a bit, or scream and gnash your teeth, or curse the gods, or whatever you need to do to express just how bad things are.

We can't ignore or worry troubling situations away. To deal with them well, we have to start by acknowledging distressing experiences as they are, without engaging defensiveness, repression, or resistance. We have to see the trouble for what it really is . . . and we have to see our reactions to trouble for what they really are.

A good way to begin the process of radical acceptance is using a tranquil practice to slow down your thoughts. You step back just enough to be able to recognize, "Right now I am having [this very troubling thought] that is causing me to feel [these troubling emotions]." Another way to jump-start radical acceptance is by using a practice that psychologist and stress researcher Elissa Epel calls the Worry Window practice.[10]

THE WORRY WINDOW

Gather several pieces of paper and something to write with. Similar to journaling, doing this longhand works better than a digital method. Then set a timer for five minutes. When you push the start button, you have only one thing to do: worry. You are creating a window in your day to worry.

Write down a few words to capture those worries. Don't censor yourself. Write down all of the big and small worries that pop up in your mind. Let your thoughts indulge in catastrophizing and exaggeration.

Your job is not to distract yourself from your worries, nor to try to explain or reason them away. Just confess them. When time is up, stop writing.

As Epel writes, "We spend a lot of time trying to rein in the mind when it starts to worry about things that haven't happened and may never happen, and that cognitive wrestling takes a toll."[11] The Worry Window eases that struggle by creating a confined time and place to fret. Another benefit of this practice is that admitting and acknowledging your worries makes them less emotionally potent. The worries probably won't go away, but they will sting a little less. In fact, studies show that creating a Worry Window reduces the amount of time you worry for the rest of the day.

Practices like the Worry Window help you admit to yourself what you are experiencing. The next step in radical acceptance is becoming more psychologically removed from those negative thoughts and feelings. This is sometimes called "distress tolerance"—gaining the ability to fully experience troubling thoughts and emotions without suppressing them or trying to explain them away. You create a mental gap between your thoughts and feelings on one hand, and your perceptions of those experiences on the other. This empowers you to be able to see those experiences, and the situations that caused them, from a more objective standpoint. In addition, you are deactivating the automatic responses you would otherwise exhibit, such as trying to push down unwanted thoughts, numbing yourself to discomfort, or engaging in behaviors to soothe yourself.[12] Self-distancing practices are highly effective for strengthening this ability. By using these practices, as Kross describes, "We can use our thoughts to change our thoughts."[13]

SELF-DISTANCING

Self-distancing is the capacity we have to step back mentally from difficult experiences, withhold an immediate response, survey the environment, and reflect on a course of action instead of being dominated by a flood of negative emotions. To gain skill with this practice, begin with an event that was emotionally difficult but not overly troubling. Recall the event and allow it to play back in your mind as if it were happening to you all over again. Focus on the feelings you were experiencing. Then, stop the recall and rest for a minute. This would be a good time to use your favorite tranquil practice.

Now, imagine that you are standing on a balcony high above that event. You are going to watch it unfold from this distant and detached perspective, as if it were a sporting event taking place on a field down below you. See yourself down on the ground in the midst of the event, but from your perspective on the balcony—it's not you down there, but another person. If you find yourself slipping into the direct experience of the event—in other words, you see yourself down on that playing field—stop, imagine yourself again on the balcony, and then let the event unfold as you watch.

Once you have replayed the entire event, write down what happened to that person down below. Yes, the person down there was you, but you watched things happen to them as if they were someone else. Use third-person pronouns to describe what happened. If you find yourself slipping into first person ("I was really scared and felt panicky"), stop and describe it again using third-person pronouns ("Matt seemed really scared and he showed signs of feeling panicky"). Describe the entire event, from beginning to end, from this neutral, third-person perspective.

After you have become skilled at using self-distancing with a moderately difficult event, you can use it with more emotionally troubling events. Researchers have found that self-distancing can be effective even with events that have caused posttraumatic stress disorder.[14]

Studies show that imagining a physical distance between yourself and a chronic stressor reduces the distress you experience. One study asked people who wanted to lose weight to imagine for ten minutes that their most tempting food was at a distance that took it out of arm's reach. If donuts were the tempting food, the participant imagined sitting in a large room with a dozen donuts at the opposite side. If pizza was the tempting food, they might imagine the pizza shop was far across town. The people who imagined distance between themselves and the tempting food were much less likely to eat that food than a control group of people who simply tried to resist the temptation.[15]

Another wise practice that builds your capacity to gain some mental distance is called Consciously Disobey Yourself, which helps strengthen your capacity to deactivate automatic responses. It fosters your ability to intentionally create a gap between your thoughts and feelings about a troubling situation, while expanding your capacity to think about them more objectively.

CONSCIOUSLY DISOBEY YOURSELF

This practice involves creating a mental disconnect between what you are thinking and what you are doing. The basic approach is to think one thing and do the opposite. Begin by using this practice with simple, everyday activities. For example, walk around a room at the same time you repeat out loud, "I cannot walk around this room." Do this for about five minutes. Or you might say out loud, "I cannot speak."

After you have practiced with everyday activities, return to your Worry Window list and select one of the stronger worries. Recall your typical response to that worry. Then, imagine a scenario where that worry would become active. Unlike the balcony practice, here you are down on the field, experiencing the troubling event. In your mind, make a statement that describes a positive response, one that is the opposite of your typical pattern. For example, "I will not go back home to check the stove, but instead reassure myself that everything is fine." Or, "I will not feel panicky, but instead I will feel strong and calm."

Although it might sound odd, this simple practice helps strengthen your capacity to disconnect from powerful thoughts and emotions that, in the past, would have swamped your capacity to respond more effectively. It won't defuse all of the distress, but it will help you be able to disconnect from the powerful surge of feelings that in the past pushed you into unhelpful responses.

The final aspect of radical acceptance is gaining a clearer and richer understanding of exactly what you are thinking and feeling. With the capacity to see your distress from a detached and distanced perspective, you can gain clarity about the content of your troubling thoughts and the nuances of the emotions you are experiencing. Practice what emotion researcher Lisa Barrett calls a highly effective way to get to know your troubling experiences better, "emotional granularity."[16]

EMOTIONAL GRANULARITY

Consider how a wine is described on its label: "This wine begins with notes of strawberry and lime, and a luscious body like soft pillows of whipped cream. As the wine sits playfully on your tongue, flavors of ripe berries evolve into . . ." You get the idea. This is how we want to describe our thoughts and emotions. Imagine that a colleague, Matt, has just said something very rude to you. Instead of thinking, *Matt's rude remark was really hurtful*, be more descriptive: *There is tightness in my chest and a burning pit in my stomach after Matt's rude remark. I feel unsafe and worried that something dangerous is lurking where I can't see it. My hands are shaky. I'm really scared.* There are many words to describe what you are feeling in more nuanced ways. The Feelings Wheel is helpful for exploring this variety (feelingswheel.com). It provides numerous shades of major emotions that can help you specify what you are experiencing.

Naming and labeling our emotions has several benefits. It helps us acknowledge them for what they are so we can then accept the reality of our experience. Like the Worry Window and self-distancing, in this description you begin to see that the rude remark made you feel that something harmful could happen again, along with a desperate need to get someplace safe. You have more insight into the nature of your experiences, which is the necessary starting point for dealing with them effectively.

Practicing emotional granularity helps you gain a finer-grained understanding of your distressing thoughts and feelings. You move from just experiencing negative emotions to actively exploring them, which creates psychological distance and allows you to detach from them. Emotional granularity also provides you with more information about what you are experiencing, which is important information for determining how to respond well to the adversity.

A study by researchers at the University of Toronto illustrates the benefits of radical acceptance.[17] They followed a group of 340 adults over six months to study the relationship between radical acceptance and wellbeing. For the first two weeks of the study, participants kept daily records of the stressors they experienced, the emotions that accompanied those experiences, and whether they responded with avoidance or acceptance. After six months, researchers assessed the participants' well-being. They found people who regularly practiced radical acceptance had lower levels of stress in response to the same kinds of stressors as the avoidance group. Acceptance was also associated with significantly higher life satisfaction and lower anxiety at the end of the study.

Radical acceptance empowers you to look at difficult situations, and the troubling thoughts and feelings they create, in ways that help you gain a clearer understanding of what's happening to you. It prepares the way for the second element of psychological flexibility, perspective taking, which is the capacity to understand the *why* of your troubling thoughts and feelings.

Perspective Taking

Most of us are "naive realists": We tend to be excessively confident in what we believe we know, and fail to recognize the full extent of our ignorance. This means that when we experience a troubling event, we cling to our initial impressions and explanations about what happened. We operate on what Nobel Prize–winning psychologist Daniel Kahneman calls the WYSIATI assumption: What You See Is All There Is.[18] We assume that our understanding of an event is 100 percent accurate. But for troubling, even awful, events, what we saw was, at best, bits and pieces of what really happened. We're unaware that our thoughts and feelings about the event are shaped by that misunderstanding. We feel worse, our thoughts get darker, and we spiral downward into distress. Things don't get better, and probably can't get better, because we are operating on faulty assumptions fueled by powerful negative emotions.

Perspective taking helps you develop more accurate understandings and insights about difficult experiences. It helps you become open minded and more willing and able to consider alternative explanations of the adversity. By taking a bigger-picture view, you can see more of what happened, especially what you missed during the initial happening and what you *thought* happened but, in fact, didn't. A good tactic to start gaining this new and helpful vantage point is to deactivate the emotions that energize the downward distress spiral. This perspective taking practice, "I Am Not My Feelings," will help stem the flow of emotional fuel to your troubling thoughts.

AFFIRMING "I AM NOT MY FEELINGS"

Thoughts and feelings are experiences you have; they are not inherent parts of who you are. You have feelings, but they don't have to have you. An important new perspective, then, is seeing that you are not your feelings. You can take the detailed descriptions from your emotional granularity practice a step further.

In this practice, make statements to yourself about the feelings you are having that affirm they are just transient experiences. Take the "Rude Matt" example again. Move away from "I feel unsafe and worried that something dangerous is lurking where I can't see it. My hands are shaky. I'm really scared," to "I am experiencing feelings that I am not safe, but they are just emotions. Emotions come and go. I *feel* scared, but fear is not part of who I am. It's just an emotion that at some point will fade away."

This is a subtle but important shift in how you see and think about disturbing experiences. When an event floods us and we feel caught in its torrential rush, we usually feel inseparably connected to the event: We *are* fear, we *are* panic. The subtle shift from thinking "I am an anxious person" to "I am a person who experiences anxiety" empowers you to see troubling thoughts and emotions as something you can handle. Rather than assuming that to overcome anxiety you have to change who you are, you recognize that you just need to attend to how you are responding to situations that cause anxious or panicky feelings. Again, this might seem like a subtle difference in perspective, but it helps you become more open minded, which is an essential part of psychological flexibility.

Shift Your Perspective

Radical acceptance empowers you to engage in perspective taking so you can see troubling events from new and more helpful viewpoints. From there, perspective shifting creates the capacity to form new and better ways of thinking and feeling about difficult experiences. Research on something called inhibitory learning explains how this happens.[19] It is really difficult to unlearn old, negative responses to difficult experiences. Those old ways are so deeply ingrained in neural pathways, it's nearly impossible to stop the negative thought pattern. You need to create new neural pathways that compete with or inhibit the automatic operation of the old, unhelpful responses. In other words, you need to create new ways for your brain to process a difficult experience. The more new pathways you create, the greater the chance your thoughts will follow a positive path.

University of Pennsylvania organizational psychologist Adam Grant writes about how to engage in perspective shifting.[20] He builds on an extensive body of research that begins with an important insight that much of our behavior is more thoughtless than thoughtful. We respond to events and people in our life without fully understanding why we are responding as we are. The key, as Grant describes it, is building the capacity to rethink:

> Part of the problem is cognitive laziness. Some psychologists point out that we're mental misers: we often prefer the ease of hanging on to old views over the difficulty of grappling with new ones. Yet there are also deeper forces behind our resistance to rethinking. Questioning ourselves makes the world more unpredictable. It requires us to admit that the facts may have changed, that what was once right may now be wrong. Reconsidering something we believe deeply can threaten our identities, making it feel as if we're losing a part of ourselves.[21]

Here's a simple example of when I recently fell headfirst into cognitive laziness. My father, my brother, and I were talking about how much one person could gift to another without incurring any taxes. My father offered one answer, but I had recently explored this topic (or so I thought) and was sure my answer was correct. I spent the day adamant that I was right. Later that night, thankfully, I felt a nudge of regret, both for my bad behavior and also because I realized I might be wrong. I went to the official Internal Revenue Service website and found my dad's answer was correct. I was wrong, by a lot. Had I taken time to rethink during that conversation, I might have been alerted to my potential mistake by the very fact that I was so dang sure I was right.

We often rely too heavily on assumptions, opinions, and past interpretations, which cloud our capacity to see problematic situations more objectively and clearly. To overcome these tendencies, Grant argues, we need to become adept at rethinking as an active, ongoing process of questioning our ideas and beliefs, being open to new information, and changing our mind when presented with better evidence or perspectives. Self-awareness is essential here. We need to be willing to examine our current assumptions, ideas, and beliefs. We also need to be aware of when we are overconfident in our thinking. It's when we feel certain, even proud, of what we "know" that we are absolutely right about that we run into problems. Becoming skillful at rethinking is a wise way to shift into a more helpful perspective.

RETHINKING

To practice rethinking, select a situation you are facing where a different perspective would be helpful. Map out how you currently think about it. What do you believe is happening? What do you think are the reasons underlying the events, interactions, and other aspects of the situation? In other words, make a list of what you think is happening and why. Be as explicit as possible about each element of your current perspective.

Work through your list, and for each element of your current perspective, find several ways you could be wrong. You will likely have to push yourself to spot these; getting other people's help is often necessary. Another way to go about this is to describe the information or evidence that would change your mind about how you are seeing the situation. This step is often the most difficult, but working through it diligently is the key to rethinking.

Then, be curious about how you might learn something new that would change how you think about the situation. You might actively invite other people to offer alternative viewpoints so you can discover ways to improve your own. Give those new ways of thinking a try. How do they change the way you understand what is happening and why it is happening? Be diligent until you arrive at a clearer understanding of the situation. Again, test your insights with other people to be sure you have, in fact, adopted a new perspective.

Another wise perspective-shifting practice is to look for the good things that might result from a problematic situation. We tend to be hyperfocused on bad outcomes, those that are happening and those we imagine might happen. This locks us into a negative perspective that constrains our capacity to think more broadly and objectively about a situation. Looking for possible silver linings can help you see new possibilities and new ways of dealing well with difficulties.

SILVER LINING PRACTICES

As the name implies, with this practice you imagine how a troubling event turns out well or produces some benefit for you or someone else.[22] Silver linings include outcomes like positive personal growth, a new relationship, or an opportunity to change your life in some favorable way. Here's an example from a close friend who has contracted Lewy body dementia: "I'm learning that there is so much more to life than my illness. That I have so many blessings that in the past I overlooked. Simple things—like a sunny day—are more special to me now."

Another silver lining practice is to imagine the helpful advice that you could give another person who experienced a similar event. This advice could help them think about the positive effects this event could have on their life, or the good things they might learn from the experience.

You can engage in preemptive silver lining practices when you are anticipating a negative experience. A study by researchers at the University of California, Riverside, explored the effects of imagining that a future stressful event would lead to positive outcomes.[23] They studied law school graduates who would soon be taking the bar exam and registered voters from both parties in advance of the 2016 presidential election. Graduates who imagined how they might grow as a person if they failed the bar exam and voters trying to focus on the good things that might happen if their preferred candidate lost reported significantly better emotional wellbeing following the actual receipt of bad news.

Habits and How They Lock Us into Problematic Responses

We sometimes get stuck responding to problematic situations in the same unhelpful way time after time. Habits, which are automatic ways of responding to a situation, are often the source of these unhelpful, repetitive responses.[24] When we are operating out of habit, we are running on autopilot and, in a very real sense, we have no perspective on the situation. We not only don't think about what we're doing, but we also often don't know why we are doing those things. We just act mindlessly. University of Southern California psychologist Wendy Wood, one of the foremost experts on habits, writes that "habits work so smoothly that we hardly ever think about them."[25]

Habits can be very helpful when they simplify daily life in positive ways. I don't have to remind myself to brush and floss at the end of the day, for example, because I am in the habit of doing both. But our deeply ingrained habits can contribute to, or even be the cause of, persistent difficulties in our life when we respond to life challenges habitually and become stuck in unhelpful ways of viewing and responding to them. Here's an example of how habits can lock people into poor responses to situations they earnestly want to change.

A group of researchers wanted to understand how eating habits of obese people might lock them into the very condition they want to change. They began the study by interviewing individuals with obesity about the difficulties they faced.[26] All of the participants expressed a sincere desire to change their eating habits but found it nearly impossible to do so. The researchers then observed these individuals at an all-you-can-eat buffet. They found that the obese eaters habitually sat facing the buffet where the food was in full view, while typical-weight diners habitually sat with their backs to the food. Typical-weight diners tended to sit in booths, where it was a bit harder to get out to go for more food, while obese eaters sat at tables in their own chairs, which made it easier. Typical-weight diners also tended to put their napkins on their laps, a small impediment to getting up for more food, whereas obese diners put theirs on the table, where they were out of the way. The biggest difference was that typical-weight diners browsed the entire buffet before making choices about what to eat, while obese diners started at the beginning of the buffet and filled their plates as they went. None of the obese eaters were aware of these habits.

Through an extensive series of studies, Wood found that all habits work through a three-phase cycle. First, an environmental cue triggers a habitual action, like seeing food at a buffet impelling people to get more. Second, those actions are repeated each time in response to that cue. This is the mindless part of a habit. Obese people get more food without thinking much about it. Cue leads to automatic response. Third, there is an immediate "reward" that follows as a result of those actions, which reinforces them. Getting more food tastes good and makes you feel full. Cue leads to automatic response that is immediately reinforced.

To change a habit, you need to address each part of the habit cycle, but the key to habit change is understanding the context in which the habit occurs and uncovering the cues that trigger it. People usually start by trying to change the automatic response, but that is very difficult to do. As Wood emphasizes, "If the context remains stable—you keep living in the same place, you keep driving the same route to work, you keep sitting on your couch every evening—then you repeat past actions automatically."[27] The response just happens, and it's nearly impossible to get out in front of it to stop it. To break a habit, you have to begin with radical acceptance about why the habit is problematic. Then, perspective taking is essential so you can spot the context cues that trigger the habit. You can then engage in perspective shifting to identify a better response.

Restoring Psychological Flexibility

When you are in the midst of chronic stress, you may find that your capacity for psychological flexibility is waning. This is normal because it is a limited resource and you may need recovery experiences to restore your reserves. Psychologist Sabine Sonnentag, a leading stress researcher, describes these as "unwinding and restoration processes" and has found that a trio of practices—detach, relax, and grow—are wise ways to restore psychological flexibility.[28]

Detachment involves finding ways to stop thinking about the stressful thing in your life for a short time. We met Carin in chapter one and learned about her struggles with chronic stress. She discovered that knitting was a detachment practice for her. As she knits, she loses track of time because she is enjoying the rhythm of the needles and the delight of seeing her project emerge. The joy of knitting helps her forget about (detach from) the stressors in her life. The key is to find something you can do that will help you not think about the difficult experiences for a little while.

Relaxation, as the name implies, helps you release the physical tension in your body. Knitting does this for Carin. She settles into a comfortable chair, turns on some quiet music, and, "as soon as I start knitting one, purling two, I am totally relaxed." Reading a good book, doing gentle stretching exercises, and using your favorite tranquil practice are also ways to relax.

Last, a growth practice is something that you really enjoy that carries with it opportunities to get better, to learn, or to in some way improve your knowledge or skill. Carin built growth into her knitting practice by taking up more sophisticated projects, like knitting a cardigan sweater using special Irish yarn. Other examples of growth practices I heard from people in my research were baking bread, playing chess, painting, gardening, and doing crossword puzzles.

Detach-relax-grow is not a solution to chronic stress. That's why you need to build psychological flexibility. But this trio can help restore and strengthen your capacities for radical acceptance, perspective taking, and perspective shifting.

Psychological flexibility is one essential for restoring and sustaining resilience. The second is adaptive coping and using wise persevering practices to strengthen and maintain it. Combining receptive practices with persevering practices will help you deal well with both everyday ups and downs and the chronic stress created by life's more troubling experiences.

KEY INSIGHTS

Building and maintaining psychological flexibility is one of the essential components of resilience. The more clearly you see things when you face troubling situations, the more effectively you manage negative thoughts and emotions.

Radical acceptance, which is one component of psychological flexibility, is the capacity to perceive and understand your thoughts and feelings about troubling situations. The more clearly you understand what you are thinking and feeling about adversity, the more effectively you can respond.

Perspective taking and perspective shifting are two more components of psychological flexibility. They help you gain the psychological distance you need both to understand what is going on in troubling situations and to see effective ways of handling them.

Detach-relax-grow practices are important during extended periods of chronic stress to restore and preserve psychological flexibility.

FURTHER READING

Insight: Why We're Not as Self-Aware as We Think, and How Seeing Ourselves Clearly Helps Us Succeed at Work and in Life by Tasha Eurich: A readable and erudite exploration of self-awareness.

Think Again: The Power of Knowing What You Don't Know by Adam Grant: Like all of his books, this one offers great illustrations and practical advice about how to break free from thinking traps.

Chatter: The Voice in Our Head, Why It Matters, and How to Harness It by Ethan Kross: A smart, accessible, highly instructive must-read guide to taming rumination.

*Overcoming Unwanted Intrusive Thoughts: A CBT-Based Guide to Getting over Frightening, Obsessive, or Disturbing Thought*s by Sally Winston and Martin N. Seif: A great read after *Chatter*, this book offers a wide range of wise practices.

Good Habits, Bad Habits: The Science of Making Positive Changes That Stick by Wendy Wood: This book offers the very best science and practical advice about habits and how to change them.

CHAPTER FIVE

Persevering Practices

Coping Well with Life Challenges

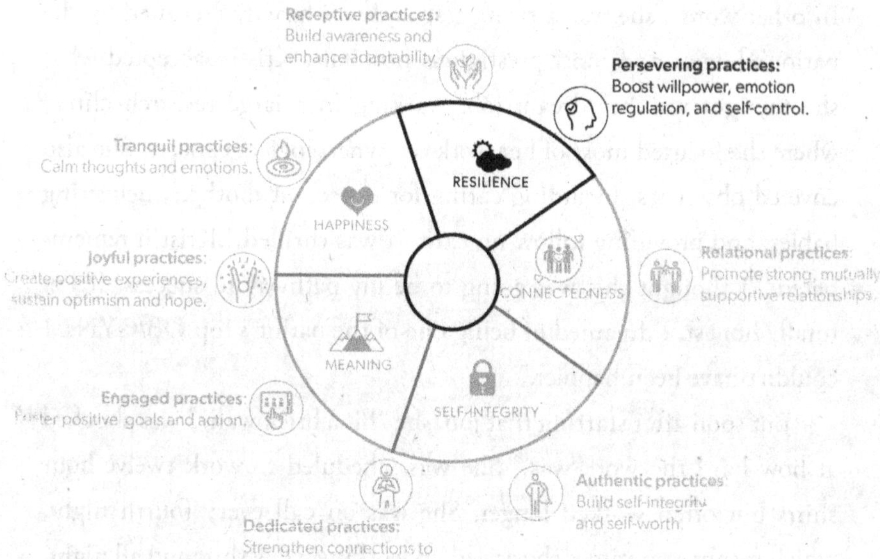

Burnout among physicians in the United States has been a significant and increasing problem over at least the past two decades.[1] Physicians experience burnout at a higher rate than the general population, and younger doctors are particularly vulnerable. I included physicians in my research to explore the work challenges they face and learn more about how physicians could sustain their wellbeing and avoid burnout. Kristin, an obstetrician-gynecologist (OB/GYN) in her forties, was one of the doctors who participated in that study. When we met, she was vibrant and energetic and loved her work. But her early experiences in medicine were far different. She had fallen into burnout but had also found a way out.

Kristin graduated from one of the top medical schools, received one of the most coveted residencies, and earned a prized fellowship. In other words, she was a rising star and was heavily recruited by the nation's largest and most prestigious hospitals. Kristin accepted what she thought was her dream job: working in a large research clinic, where she focused most of her work on gynecological cancers. She also covered obstetrics, including caring for expectant mothers, delivering babies, and providing follow-up care. "I was thrilled," Kristin remembered. "I thought this was going to be my pathway to success. If I'm totally honest, I dreamed of being one of the nation's top OB/GYNs. I couldn't have been happier."

But soon after starting that job, she "hit a brick wall. I was shocked at how hard the work was." She was scheduled to work twelve-hour shifts but often worked longer. She was on call every fourth night, which meant sometimes she ended up working a day shift and all night, twenty-four hours or more in a row. She faced heavy pressure to care for a quota of patients, which meant she was often hectically rushing from one to another with no time even for bathroom breaks. "Most nights I collapsed on my bed too exhausted to eat," Kristin said. "I slept a few hours, managed to choke down some breakfast, then trudged back to the clinic." There were also intense pressures to do work that could be published in top medical journals, but "I was so tired and worried that I wasn't able to come up with any ideas. Some of the senior researchers seemed to have dozens of publishable projects and I couldn't even come up with one."

Kristin's initial reaction was to keep going. "I thought I just needed to adjust. It was new to me, and I just needed to adapt to that pace of work. I thought that I just needed to push through and the only way to do that is to keep going, keep trying, grind it out." And she did. Or, that's what she tried to do. "I have always been a hard worker, and so there was a certain amount of pride, I guess, that I should be able to push through," she told me. "Looking back, I think I just didn't want to fail and I was willing to pay whatever it cost to succeed." So, she kept pushing, kept worrying that she was failing, and kept feeling more and more exhausted.

The stress built up until one day she couldn't get out of bed. "It wasn't that I was very tired and dreaded work," she said, "it was that I physically was unable to stand up." She crawled to the bathroom, vomited, drank some water, and collapsed on the floor. Several hours later she woke up, got up, ate a light meal, and went to work. The next day it happened again. Kristin called her boyfriend, who cared for her for the three days it took to regain her strength. "I was mortified that I had to call in sick for even one day. Three seemed unforgivable." She had all of the classic symptoms of raging burnout, but like many of her colleagues, she pushed on. "The chief of my clinic had told me several times that I needed to figure things out. Finally, he suggested I take a leave of absence, which would have been a huge career hit. I couldn't do that." A year later, after several more bouts of extreme exhaustion, and with a deep sense of despair, she quit, thinking her medical career was over. "I just couldn't go on. It's hard to convey how desperate and difficult that was. I felt like I was giving up everything: my career, my dream, my identity because I felt being a doctor was what I was meant to do."

Fast-forward to the time of our interview. After quitting, Kristin took a year off work to regain her physical health and wellbeing. She then took a job at a smaller hospital in its OB/GYN clinic. "Making a dramatic change in my working conditions was a difficult decision, but I knew it was essential," she reported. "Plus, it was a chance to be a doctor again. It has turned out to be one of the most important career decisions I have made."

Perhaps even more essential were the wise wellbeing practices Kristin had learned during her year away from work, and continued when she started work again. Speaking about those practices, she said, "They are foundational to my mental health. I've learned that doing them regularly keeps me healthy. They allow me to do the work I love." Kristin has a daily tranquil practice: "I do contemplative prayer every day. I never, ever miss. It only takes fifteen to twenty minutes, but it grounds and calms me. I can even do it at the clinic if I have to be there extra early." Kristin also learned to use diligent practices, including how to distance herself from stressful situations. "I've learned how to avoid becoming emotionally immersed when something bad happens, like when a cancer patient dies or a baby is in extreme distress. I can detach myself. I still care a lot about my patients, but I've learned to step back emotionally from those experiences. I can respond more effectively as a physician. And I don't carry those situations home with me anymore." Over time, Kristin has added in other wise practices. "I exercise regularly. You'd be surprised about how many physicians don't. One of the benefits of that is I no longer let the stress of work build up."

Another wise practice Kristin adopted early and continues to use is changing her situations when she can. "Early on in my time at [the new clinic] I accepted every on-call duty I was assigned. Then I realized that was not sustainable: I was falling back into the same bad habits. I had a talk with [the chief medical officer] about it and told him I could only be on call once a week. This was less than some of my male colleagues, and I worried about being labeled 'weak.' But it turned out great. The chief decided to re-evaluate call for everyone. Now, all of the physicians have better call schedules. A couple of my male colleagues even thanked me for being brave enough to raise the issue."

At the time she experienced burnout, Kristin didn't know that many other physicians, both those new to medicine and those who had been practicing for years, had had similar experiences. A 2024 study of physician wellbeing found that almost half of doctors were experiencing at least one symptom of severe burnout.[2] Another physician told me, "Doctors sometimes don't want to admit they're human, that they have limits. And the professional culture tells us we are weak, failures, if we can't deal with work and stress. I remember that in the Bible Jesus says, 'Physician, heal thyself.' That's what we need to do, heal ourselves so we can heal others. But most of us don't."

Throughout my research and my teaching MBA students and executives, I heard similar stories from many people across professions. Troubling situations like dealing with demanding work, having a difficult boss, grieving a significant loss, holding things together as you race toward a big deadline, coping with a major health challenge, or juggling an over-full schedule are very common, and these can create chronic stress that taxes your resilience and can undermine your wellbeing. Like Kristin in her early career, many of us default to avoidance tactics: We ignore the situation, try to push troubling thoughts and emotions out of our mind, or cling to the hope that things will get better. If we try to grind it out, too often we get ground up as a result. Avoidance only makes things worse.[3]

Persevering practices build your capacity for adaptive coping and empower you to deal effectively with adversity in three ways. These practices help sustain and strengthen willpower, which is the capacity to control your impulses, manage your behavior, and persist in the face of adversity. Persevering practices also help you adopt a challenge orientation toward adversity so that you view it as a problem you can overcome rather than a threat you must avoid. Last, persevering practices enhance your capacity to express negative thoughts and emotions in more constructive ways.

Take another look at the graphic at the start of this chapter. Remember that the five dimensions of wellbeing are deeply connected, intertwined like the parts of our physical health. They build on, reinforce, and depend on each other. We need all of them to be at sufficient levels (i.e., scoring at least a 7 on each dimension of the wellbeing assessment). Well, wise practices are also interconnected. This is especially true with receptive and persevering practices. They work together and build on each other. If resilience is an area of need for you, start by integrating a receptive practice or two into your daily life, then build on that by adding in one or more persevering practices. A good place to start is a wise practice that will strengthen your willpower, so let's take a look at the science of how that works.

Willpower

All coping is fueled by our willpower. Psychologist Roy Baumeister, the leading researcher of willpower, describes it using what he calls the muscle metaphor. Imagine for a moment a good friend has asked you to help them move apartments (groan!). On the day of the move, you carry box after box from the old apartment to the moving truck, then from the truck into the new apartment. By the end of the day, your arm and leg muscles are exhausted. Willpower is like that: When you have to exert a lot of self-control to, for example, avoid temptations, control your anger, or stay focused on a task, the strength of your willpower muscle is temporarily depleted.

Here's a classic study of willpower depletion.[4] Participating students were ushered into a lab where the smell of freshly baked chocolate chip cookies filled the room. They sat down at a table with several food choices: chocolate chip cookies, some pieces of chocolate, and a bowl of radishes. Half of these students were placed in a control group and were invited to eat the cookies and chocolate right away. The other half were told to only eat radishes and leave the cookies and chocolate alone. The researchers left students in both groups alone for about five minutes and observed them behind a one-way mirror. Not surprisingly, the students in the control group gobbled up the sweets. Those in the radish-only group were clearly tempted by the cookies and chocolate. Most looked intensely at the treats; several picked up a cookie and smelled it. But none of the radish-only students gave in to temptation.

Then, both groups were taken into another room and asked to solve puzzles to "test their cleverness." The puzzles were really unsolvable; it was a test of how long they would persist before giving up. The radish-only group quit, on average, within eight minutes, while the cookies and chocolate group worked, on average, for twenty minutes. This was one of the first studies to show that using your willpower temporarily depletes your capacity to exercise it. Since then, dozens of studies have demonstrated the depleted-muscle effect.

Just as you can make a muscle stronger through proper exercise, you can strengthen your willpower. The more you use it, the stronger your mental muscle becomes. Making time for the right kind of workout is a good way to build a more powerful willpower muscle.

WILLPOWER WORKOUTS

One of the best ways to strengthen your willpower is to practice using it on important but simple tasks. For example, you might work on your posture by sitting up straight each time you catch yourself slouching. You first set a clear intention for why you want to sit up straight rather than slouch, something straightforward like "I want to have good posture because it's better for my back." Then, set another intention of reminding yourself of this every time you slouch. When you catch yourself slouching, sit up straight! You're working out your willpower muscle.

Another willpower workout might be changing your speech habits by getting rid of verbal fillers such as "like," "uh," and "you know." Again, begin with a clear intention of why you want to do this, and then an intention that you will stop yourself from using those fillers. A third example is doing routine tasks like eating or brushing your teeth with your alternative hand. Or, change your routine such as making your bed every day if you don't already do so, or praying three times a day, or tidying your workspace at the end of each day.

The basic form of this practice is to introduce a small change in some routine part of your daily life that will require using your willpower.

When willpower reserves are depleted, we are much more likely to fall back on automatic responses. I saw an example of this recently while I was waiting in line to order some ice cream. The two people in front of me were talking about how much they love ice cream but also their strong desire to eat healthy and control their weight. They spoke about "not wanting to order too much," but both walked away with triple-scoop sundaes with lots of trimmings. I don't know how they spent their day before the ice cream order—they both had on logo shirts that indicated they had been working—but I bet it was full of willpower-depleting tasks.

Given that willpower is a limited resource, it is important to learn the signs that your willpower muscle is tiring, what I call your willpower tells. Poker players describe how some people unwittingly "tell" when they have a good or bad hand. It might be wiping their forehead when they don't have good cards or smiling subtly when they have a strong hand. Learning about your willpower tells prepares you to make better choices about how to respond in an adaptive way. It will also alert you to when you need restoration practices to reenergize your willpower muscle.

KNOW YOUR WILLPOWER TELLS

This practice is another adaptation of Map Your Days. Have a piece of paper and pen, or calendar, or some other writing surface and tool handy throughout the day. At several times throughout the day, say ten o'clock, two, and four, pause to rate how stressful and busy your day is. Very quickly rate the day with something like 1 (*easy day, no stress*) to 5 (*intensely stressful*). Or use a smiley, neutral, or frowny face for an easy, normal, or very busy day. Then take a minute to quickly scan your body and notice any place you feel tense or uncomfortable. Note also your emotions and describe what you are feeling.

Do this for several days, longer if you can, then look back over the daily events, bodily feelings, and emotions you experienced. Take note of the signs that indicated your willpower was dwindling. Look for patterns, then take those insights into the next week. Do the same thrice-daily quick self-examination, but look through the lens of the insights you found in the first part of the practice. You will begin to see some of your willpower tells. Mine begin with tension in my upper back and neck. For years I never noticed this, but now I am more keenly aware of that tension. I also feel more irritable and impatient. At first these symptoms are mild, but because I have used this practice several times, I can now sense them when they are first showing up.

A study led by researchers at Maastricht University in the Netherlands illustrates how stressful situations can weaken your willpower muscle.[5] For two weeks they had 135 working adults keep a diary similar to the one I just described. In the morning, at midday, and in the afternoon, participants recorded how aversive or demanding their work tasks were and how "mentally" strong or depleted they felt. In the afternoon, they rated the strength of their willpower and their work performance for that day. The results indicated that the more demanding that work had been in the morning, the greater the reduction in participants' willpower and performance later in the day.

There was an additional interesting part to the study. Participants also recorded how often they rewarded themselves during a difficult day. They responded yes or no to "This morning/afternoon, I rewarded myself with something special." People who used self-rewards experienced less willpower depletion and, as a result, better performance. The study did not capture what these self-rewards were, but it suggests that being kind to yourself on difficult days can help keep your willpower muscle stronger.

Adopt a Challenge Orientation

In chapter four on receptive practices, we learned how shifting our perspective can help us view difficult situations in more positive and helpful ways and help us respond to adversity better. Columbia University psychologist George Bonanno, an expert on resilience, describes our typical orientation:

> When people are confronted with serious adversity, it is only natural to feel threatened and, at least initially, to focus on how bad things might get . . . In essence, we are telling ourselves, "This is going to be bad, and it will probably get worse. I don't

think I can handle it." The more we stay focused on the threat, the more likely we are to become distressed and anxious. Distressing, anxious emotions, in turn, often get in the way of our ability to take effective action.[6]

His research documents the importance of shifting to a challenge orientation, an extension of the "stress is enhancing" perspective, in which you view the troubling situation as something you can handle and that might even help you grow stronger and more capable of dealing with future hardships. When we view the situation as a challenge, as Bonanno writes,

> we take a more active stance, and we begin to think about the stressor differently. We see it less as a threat to endure and more as a challenge to be met. In other words, when we embrace a challenge, we shift from simply telling ourselves how bad it is going to be to focusing on what we need to do to get past it.[7]

This subtle but important shift operates in at least two ways. First, it changes your semantic information processing, which means it shapes the things you notice and the interpretations you make of those things. Rather than seeing events as sources of threat and danger, you see them as problems you can do something about. Instead of seeing yourself as helpless, you see the strengths and capacities you have to act effectively. Second, it creates a positive bias in your thinking. You notice opportunities to make things better and feel eager to work toward them, leaning in to the problematic situation rather than running away from it.

Our social culture and media outlets portray stress as always a bad and potentially very detrimental experience. But Hans Selye, who conducted pioneering research on stress, distinguished between forms that are detrimental, what he called "distress," and "eustress," forms of stress that catalyze performance and growth. Think of an Olympic sprinter in the blocks just before the starting gun, a singer about to go on stage before thousands of fans, or a student who has just been handed a college entrance exam. All three likely feel a surge of energy, and probably some nervousness, from stress because they see their situations as a challenge. Because they see stress as enhancing their capacity to perform, they feel full of energy and strongly motivated to perform well. We experience eustress in many situations, like when we are getting married, having a baby, starting a new job, gearing up for a school or work presentation, making a new friend, going out on a first date, or leaving for a vacation.

ADOPT A "STRESS IS ENHANCING" MINDSET

This practice begins with radical acceptance: acknowledging and owning the stress you feel. The next step is to recognize that all stress arises because something you care about is at stake. Perhaps it is performance on an important project, or the safety of someone you love, or a desire to be healthier. Take time to imagine yourself welcoming the stress because it reflects something you care about. Ask yourself, "Am I feeling stressed about this because I really care about ________?" Identifying this underlying positive need or goal helps create a positive mindset about stress.

The final step is to imagine how you can use the stress response positively. For example, remembering that stress energizes you, visualize how it is preparing your mind and body to take action. Imagine that your stress means you are excited and ready for a challenge, rather than scared or unprepared. Look for the opportunities that arise because of, not in spite of, the stress, like developing a new skill or strengthening a relationship by relying on another person for help. This step may require stretching your imagination, so take your time with it. You can also ask other people to help you identify the opportunities the stressful situation has created.

Stanford University psychologist Alia Crum studied how seeing stress as a positive challenge can enhance your capacity to respond well. In a series of studies with over seven hundred working adults, Crum and her colleagues divided participants into two groups: One would receive training on how to shift to a "stress is enhancing" perspective, and the other was put on a waitlist for future training.[8] Four weeks after, both groups were asked a series of questions about their physical health and wellbeing. Compared to people on the waitlist, trained participants "reported reductions in self-reported negative health symptoms associated with stress and anxiety; better performance at work with respect to generating new ideas, sustaining focus, being engaged, and collaborating well with others; and greater overall satisfaction with their health."[9] Other studies have confirmed these kinds of positive outcomes from shifting to a more positive perspective on stress.

Adopting a challenge orientation also helps you override automatic processing and stay out of the downward distress spiral. Instead of reacting, you choose how to act. And responding intentionally to adversity is the deeper shift we are after. Another way to adopt a challenge orientation is to change the way you talk to yourself about adversity. You might say to yourself, "The future will be okay," or "I have the capacity to handle the challenges I face." Simple statements like these remind you to take an active stance toward adversity.

A final way to shift to a challenge orientation is by using self-distancing practices.

DISTANCED SELF-TALK

Our inner monologue tends to be from our own perspective. "I am sick and tired of being treated so poorly" and "I am really worried I will bomb that speech" are examples of how we talk to ourselves about difficult events in ways that are threat oriented. Research on self-talk shows that by changing the perspective of our inner talk, we can shift to a challenge mindset.

To practice, recall a moderately difficult or troubling recent experience. As you replay it in your mind, play the part of a narrator or (if you're a sports fan) a play-by-play announcer. Describe that experience in as much detail as you can using your name and third-person pronouns. As you work through the experience, describing it as if the person going through it were not you, pause from time to time and ask questions like "What is Matt doing, and why is he doing those things?" "What does Matt seem to be feeling, and why does he feel this way?" "What is he thinking?" and "What are the underlying causes of Matt's feelings and thoughts?"

When you have worked your way through the entire experience, take a moment to reflect on the questions you asked and jot down notes about the thoughts and insights that are emerging. It might take several times running through the play-by-play for insights to crystallize. Then, again using third-person language, identify and describe the opportunities "Matt" (in my case) had to view the experience as a challenge. Look for places where the person could have used the situation to gain new self-knowledge, achieve personal growth, or lean on the support of other people. Practicing with several moderately difficult experiences will help you gain skill in using this practice on more serious or distressing life events.

Researcher Ethan Kross and his colleagues showed that distanced self-talk led people to spontaneously take on a challenge orientation.[10] They studied people who had to give a speech they initially described as "nerve-racking." Those who were trained to use this self-talk practice and then asked to describe how they were thinking about the speech shifted to a challenge mindset without additional prompting. For example, one participant described it this way: "First, I asked myself what was I nervous about? It's not like this will be the first interview or speech I've ever had to give. And even if it doesn't go perfectly, it won't be the end of the world. I'll learn something that will help me be better at public speaking." Another said, "I told myself that I'm not under a lot of pressure for this. I'm qualified and have worked hard; I have confidence in my abilities."

A challenge orientation is especially important when adversity persists over time. Studying the mindsets of people who suffered spinal cord injuries, Bonanno found that those who adopted a challenge orientation were much less likely to become depressed, tended to adopt an "I won't let this ruin my life" attitude, and over time developed a new sense of meaning and purpose in life. Even though their physical condition did not improve, they were happier and more satisfied. His research also demonstrated that wise practices can be highly effective nudges for people who have experienced dramatic shocks to their well-being, like spinal cord injuries. Imagine, then, how this change in orientation might help with the difficulties you face.

Express Thoughts and Emotions Constructively

Adversities tend to amp up negative emotions and trigger distressing thoughts. Wise practices can help you express negative emotions constructively while fostering positive thoughts and feelings.[11] Given that we tend to be unaware of our historic pattern of responses to troublesome situations, stepping back to review recent reactions to adversity can provide insights into how you typically respond and what kinds of adversity trigger particular responses. This is a way of developing the capacity to "know before," as I described in chapter four. With that knowledge, you can prepare yourself to respond more adaptively by, for example, imagining yourself engaging in more adaptive responses.

TAKING A COPING INVENTORY

Begin by reflecting on the past year or so, then write down all of the moderately to severely problematic or troubling experiences you faced. For each experience, briefly describe what it was about (e.g., a disagreement with your partner, a stressful deadline, the death of your mother), what you thought and felt at the time of the event, and how you handled it. Then make an honest assessment of how things turned out, especially how well you dealt with each situation. You are creating a list of coping tactics that work well for you and those that don't. This isn't a time for sharp self-criticism; it's an opportunity to step back and learn from past experience.

Here's an example: I agreed to give a speech in two months. At first, I worried and stewed about it. I woke up at night thinking about it, trying to work out what I would say. Then, one day I decided to make an outline of the speech. The outline was incomplete, but it helped me see I would be able to prepare well. I put the outline away until two weeks before the event and didn't think much about it until then. I had plenty of time to prepare and felt confident about what I would say. And the speech seemed to go well.

By looking back over your list, you can identify the tactics that worked best for you and the situations for which they were most effective. It's also a good way to start boosting your confidence in your capacity to manage your thoughts and emotions because you see where you have responded well!

Sometimes you can modify an adverse situation to help you respond adaptively. Using contextual nudges is one approach. People who are struggling to lose weight, for example, can use smaller plates and bowls to encourage them to take smaller portions. They can get rid of problematic food in their home, place healthy snacks in easy-to-grab places, plan meals that are both tasty and nutritious, and eat as often as possible with people who will affirm and encourage them.

From my coping inventory, I learned that arriving at a speaking venue just before I went on stage amped up my nervousness, which caused me to worry about all kinds of things: Did I remember my laptop with my slides? Am I dressed appropriately? Will I remember what I want to say? I changed my pattern and began arriving before the audience filed in. I walked around the venue to become more familiar and comfortable with my surroundings. I asked for a lapel microphone because my hands sometimes shook with a handheld one, which made me more nervous. I had the podium removed because I am more at ease walking when I speak. And, whenever possible, I didn't wear a suit coat and tie, because I am uncomfortable in them. Over time, those simple changes helped me feel at ease and confident. I rarely worry ahead of time, and on the day of, I am self-assured and eager to share what I know.

As another example, there was a time when Kim and I needed to set a spending budget, but we simply couldn't stick to one. We worried a lot about how we were going to get control of our finances. Kim learned about a situation-change technique that worked for us. We got cash for all of our expenses,, back when cash was still widely used. We labeled a set of jars with our expenses: "house payment," "food," "credit card bill," and so on—one jar for each monthly expense. We also had an "entertainment" jar, which we filled last because that category was usually our budget buster. We drew from that jar at the end of each week as a reward for sticking with the budget jars. It worked; within a year we were debt free.

Another situation-change practice that I used when I was in the middle of a difficult time at work was to end my day on a high note. It helped me build some positivity into really tough days so I could respond in more adaptive and helpful ways.

END ON A HIGH NOTE

Research shows that when we remember an experience, the way it ends has a significant effect on that memory. Furthermore, a positive ending makes an otherwise difficult experience less stressful. Knowing something about what makes your days good and bad is a necessary starting place, so this is another practice that can build on Map Your Days. When I was a professor, grading days were really stressful. Having taken the time to map my days, I knew that meeting with students was almost always a high-point experience. So, on grading days, whenever possible I ended my day by meeting with a student. Grading still weighed heavy, but ending on a high note made those days much less taxing.

To end on a high note, you need to do three things: Figure out what your high-note experiences are, plan how to work them into the end of your day, and form a clear intention of when and how you will end your days with them. For example, I walked to and from work, so after a tough day I would listen to inspiring music like Aaron Copland's *Fanfare for the Common Man* or U2's *The Joshua Tree* album on the walk home.

Other times, to cope adaptively we need to physically release what we are feeling. Maybe when you are really frustrated or angry, screaming into a pillow is helpful. A vigorous physical workout, like high-intensity interval training, works well for me when I am feeling mad, irritated, or worried. Kim has invented her own practice to vent negative feelings, which she calls Boo-Hoo Movies.

BOO-HOO MOVIES

Sometimes, the best way to respond better is to allow your emotions and thoughts to flow temporarily. When Kim has been feeling a lot of pent-up emotions and needs a way to let them out, she watches a tear-jerker movie. The sadness and grief she experiences while watching help her release the flow—more often the flood—of suppressed emotions. When she is "all cried out," Kim feels unburdened, refreshed, and ready to deal with the underlying cause of those emotions.

Comedian and actor Margaret Cho shared with me that watching horror movies creates a similar release for her. She says that when she is feeling fearful or especially worried, seeing an externalized expression of fear helps her release her pent-up emotions. The "horror out there" allows her to detach and even process the "horror in here."

One pastor I interviewed said that singing hymns as loud as he could was a great way to shed negative feelings. A group of humanitarian workers would turn on loud music and "dance like maniacs" when they were in the middle of emotionally charged situations. A schoolteacher would bang a drum as loud and as hard as she could after a tough day at work.

These kinds of practices can help when we are in the middle of a troubling situation. But how can you deal with feelings from past adversity? Expressive writing, a practice developed by University of Texas psychologist James Pennebaker, can be a highly effective coping practice for a variety of past experiences, including those that create posttraumatic stress disorder.[12] I've learned that it works best if I take my time and spread the phases out over several days.

EXPRESSIVE WRITING

There are four phases to this practice. Take as long as you need to complete each phase. Writing each day if possible can be helpful, and you can spread writing on each phase over several days. When you finish each writing session, do something restorative: Engage in a relaxing or enjoyable activity, spend time with family or friends, or use a tranquil practice.

Phase I is "pour it out." Write about the emotionally troubling event and what you experienced. Write in the first person, and don't hold back or censor yourself. Your goal is to write fully about what you experienced, especially your thoughts and feelings. Try to write for at least twenty minutes, but take as long as you need. Write continuously, with few or no interruptions. You can repeat this phase several times if it will help you really pour it out.

Phase II is "step back." Describe your experience from an objective viewpoint, writing as someone who just observed what you went through, like a news reporter, and is now describing that experience. As you have done in other practices, write in the third person. Describe the place and location where the event happened. Record the event in a step-by-step manner, writing about the other people involved, what they did, and how they responded. Then, report on the implications of this event for the focal person (you). How did it affect them? What were their responses?

Phase III is "write a story." Return to writing in the first person and create a structured storyline about your experience that has a clear beginning, middle, and end. This is often the phase during which people are able to "process" their experience in a helpful way. Write about how the event began, which might require telling the story of events that led up to the focal experience. Then, write about the experience itself. As you write, do your best to create a plot line for your story. Write about what caused you to think or feel a certain way. Write about why things happened as they did. Create a clear ending: "This is how the event came to its conclusion." Finish your story by writing about the insights you gained about yourself or the lessons you can take away from the experience, and then write about the silver linings that followed from it. You might have to look hard for these, but finding something good that followed from the adversity will be important. Rewrite your story until you are bored with it; being bored is a good indicator that you have processed the story fully.

Phase IV is "imagine a better future." This phase is optional, but it can be very helpful. Write about a new future in which the troubling experience changed you for the better. Write about how you have grown as a result of that experience. You might describe the things you have learned from that event or how you would respond differently to a similar emotionally troubling event in the future.

You can also use expressive writing for present or future events like relationship problems, major life transitions like deciding whether to leave a stressful job or losing a loved one, and positive but complicated events like starting a new job or becoming a new parent.

Expressive writing is an especially wise and helpful practice. Because it comprises both receptive and persevering practices, it can help you remember how psychological flexibility and adaptive coping work. In phase I you are engaging in radical acceptance, and in phase II you are using perspective taking and shifting. In phases III and IV you are using a wise adaptive coping practice.

KEY INSIGHTS

- Adaptive coping, the second essential component of resilience, is your ability to deal well with the ups and downs of life, and your capacity to face and overcome adversities with skill and equanimity. Over time, pursuing its combination of receptive and persevering practices will build your capacity to deal well with almost anything that comes your way.
- Willpower—the ability to manage your thoughts, feelings, and actions—is the essential psychological capacity that powers resilience. Persevering practices restore and sustain willpower.
- Adopting a challenge orientation, where you see difficulties as challenges you can overcome, rather than threats you need to avoid, enhances your capacity to respond constructively.
- Learning constructive ways to express negative thoughts and feelings rather than letting them build up or expressing them in maladaptive ways is also an important part of adaptive coping.

FURTHER READING

The End of Trauma: How the New Science of Resilience Is Changing How We Think About PTSD by George A. Bonanno: An instructive guide written by one of the world's foremost experts on resilience.

Permission to Feel: Unlocking the Power of Emotions to Help Our Kids, Ourselves, and Our Society Thrive by Marc Brackett: A very helpful exploration of the science of emotions, and how it can help you become skillful at regulating them.

A Liberated Mind: How to Pivot Toward What Matters by Steven C. Hayes: Part memoir, part science-based instruction guide, this book is one of the best guides to radical acceptance and perspective shifting.

The Body Keeps the Score: Brain, Mind, and Body in the Healing of Trauma by Bessel van der Kolk: An amazing and revelatory book on stress, resilience, and trauma.

Hope for Cynics: The Surprising Science of Human Goodness by Jamil Zaki: If the news makes you feel hopeless, this book will give you a path to find hope again.

CHAPTER SIX

Relational Practices

Nurturing Strong Social Support

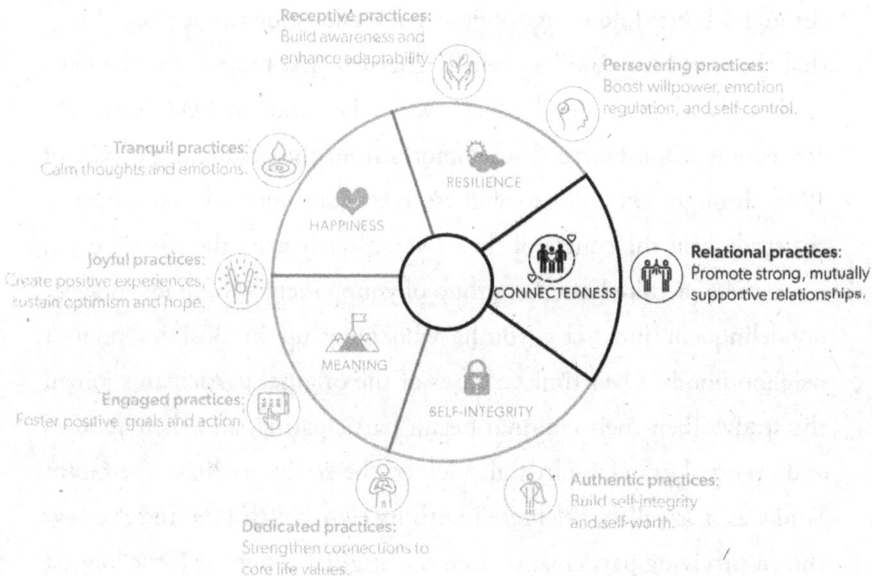

In 1936 William T. Grant was a tycoon.[1] Thirty years earlier he'd opened a single "25 cent store," then opened more stores as he prospered. His "Grant's Stores," as customers called them, were brick-and-mortar predecessors to Amazon that sold clothes, toys, home goods, furniture, electronics, and more. Grant's mission was to offer "great value to customers at a modest price." People responded enthusiastically. At the height of the Great Depression, his company had several hundred stores and was worth $100 million, the equivalent of almost $2 billion in 2025 dollars. It made Grant one of the wealthiest people in the United States.

Grant decided to share his wealth, so in 1936 he created a foundation to advance research in the social sciences. "What I have in mind," he wrote, "is to assist, by some means, in helping people or peoples to live more contentedly and peacefully and well in body and mind through a better knowledge of how to use and enjoy all the good things that the world has to offer them."[2] The very first project was the Harvard Study of Adult Development, which launched in 1938. Researchers recruited 268 Harvard sophomores from the graduating classes of 1942 through 1944. Most of these men continued to participate in the study over the course of their lives. Shortly after the study began, researchers recruited another group of young men: 456 disadvantaged, nondelinquent inner-city youths who grew up in Boston's poorest neighborhoods. Over time, spouses of the original participants joined the study. Then their children began participating, and their spouses and eventual grandchildren also joined the study. In 2024, the Grant Study, as it is called, celebrated both its eighty-fifth year and the seventeen surviving participants from the original cohort. It is the longest study of wellbeing in history.[3]

Researchers began with a very comprehensive assessment of each young man. The first medical exam evaluated major organ function, assessed lactic acid levels during treadmill tests, gathered electroencephalographs of participants' brain activity, and measured nearly every dimension of their bodies, including the hanging length of their scrotums. Psychiatrists held lengthy meetings with each man to collect thorough life histories. Topics included when a participant stopped wetting the bed, how he learned about sex, and a comprehensive mapping of key past and present social relationships. Participants also took a battery of psychological tests including intelligence tests, Rorschach inkblot interpretations, and handwriting analysis. Social workers interviewed students' parents to gather more data about their home life and childhood. Every two years the "Grant men" participated in extensive physical and psychological examinations. Researchers gathered data over time about personal habits (living situation, daily activities, smoking, alcohol consumption), social relationships (quality of marriage, family relationships, friendships, parenting), work and careers (job and income, typical work activities and responsibilities, work satisfaction and stress), and major life events (marriage, divorce, serious illness or injury, job change, loss of loved ones).

Like the Framingham Heart Study, this project produced many groundbreaking discoveries. Because its data have been gathered on the same people over many decades, its most important insights include science-based understandings of the keys to living a long, happy, healthy, fulfilling life. These include refraining from smoking and overuse of alcohol, adapting well to life challenges and changes, and maintaining an active lifestyle.

But the research team discovered that one factor is, far and away, the most important for a lifetime of wellbeing. The study's current director, Robert Waldinger, sums up that discovery this way: "If we had to take all eighty-five years of the Grant Study and boil it down to a single principle for living, one life investment that is supported by similar findings across a variety of other studies, it would be this: Good relationships keep us healthier and happier."[4]

Because the Grant Study followed participants into their eighties, researchers were able to look back at each participant's historical data to see what predicted those who became happy, healthy octogenarians and those who didn't. It wasn't their wealth, or the prestige of their jobs, or their middle-aged cholesterol levels that mattered most, although all of these were important; it was having warm, caring relationships over their life course. And not just good relationships with family and friends; relationships with coworkers and bosses, neighbors, and others in their social ecosystem also mattered.

Hundreds of other research studies confirm that strong, caring, supportive relationships are one of the most important factors for building and sustaining both health and wellbeing.[5] We need to know that other people know, value, and care about us. We need people we can depend on in the best times and in the most difficult times. We need to feel valued and validated by others. And we need these kinds of relationships in all the major areas of our lives: at home, in social contexts, and at work.

Of particular importance are our relationships with significant and similar others. Significant others include our spouses and partners, close family and friends, and other people who provide love and care for us. Similar others are people who fill comparable social roles to our own—for example, people with the same job, who are also parents of young children, or who are members of the same ethnic group. They are also those with whom we share significant core characteristics (e.g., being an introvert) and life experiences (e.g., similar childhoods, shared traumatic experiences). Similar others are uniquely positioned to commiserate with us during difficult times and celebrate genuinely with us in good times because of these similar roles or experiences. They can provide personalized advice when we face challenges and the right kind of encouragement when we need a boost. Relational practices promote and sustain strong, mutually supportive social relationships. These practices help us develop new relationships, strengthen existing ones, and mend broken ones.

The structure of this chapter is a bit different from the others. I will first share the core characteristics of good relationships. With those essential characteristics in mind, we will then explore how to build and sustain them. And, of course, every practice in this chapter is also a great way to step together. Spoiler alert: The most important research insight herein is that the key to sustaining strong, positive relationships is to always be a relationship builder. Relationships, of course, require at least two people to actively engage. But someone has to start, either to begin a relationship, to make it stronger, or to repair it. So, be the first to build and always be a builder.

What We Need from Relationships

The five core characteristics of all good relationships are that all parties feel known, respected, safe, valued, and supported. These characteristics are essential for relationships with someone we will likely see only once, such as a restaurant server or flight attendant; with someone at work, like a client or colleague; and with friends, family members, and life partners. Of course, the way each of these characteristics shows up varies with each relationship, but all of them matter for any connections we have with another person. They work together to form the foundational structure of good relationships.

Here's a quick metaphor. Imagine that you have five different colors of Play-Doh: red, blue, green, orange, and purple. You mash and roll the five pieces together into a rough ball. When you look at the ball, you can see bits of the individual colors, but most of it is a blend of colors. These five characteristics work like that by forming the Play-Doh ball of good relationships. They are mutually reinforcing: As one characteristic grows deeper, the others also deepen. For example, the better we get to know another person, and the more they know about us, the more they affirm who we are and the closer we feel to them.

I hope this chapter will encourage you to recognize and appreciate the variety of relationships you have. You might begin with a wise practice used in the Grant Study called Your Relationship Universe.[6]

MAPPING YOUR RELATIONSHIP UNIVERSE

You will need paper and a writing instrument for this practice. Make a big plus sign (+) in the middle of the paper, large enough to almost fill it. On the horizontal line, mark the left end with "Infrequent" and the right with "Very Frequent." This denotes how often you interact with a particular person. On the vertical line, mark the top with "Energizing" and the bottom with "Depleting." As Waldinger and Marc Schulz, his colleague in the project, describe,

"An energizing relationship enlivens and invigorates you, and it gives you a sense of connection and belonging that remains after the two of you part ways. It makes you feel better than you would feel if you were alone . . . A depleting relationship induces tension, frustration, or anxiety, and makes you feel worried, or even demoralized. In some ways, it makes you feel lesser or more disconnected than you would feel if you were alone."[7]

Now you have four quadrants or spaces to fill. Begin with the upper right, "Energizing and Very Frequent." Here you can place the people you are closest to and that you see most often. I would put Kim, my father, my sons, my daughter-in-law, my brothers, and a few others. These are my people! You might then move to the upper left corner, "Energizing and Infrequent." I would put my friends Michael, Dan, John, Steve, and Joe here. You can also add in groups, so I would put my scuba-diving buddies in this quadrant. Then move to the lower right quadrant—these are your most difficult relationships, because you have frequent, depleting interactions with these people. Last, fill in the lower left corner with your infrequent, depleting contacts. The finished chart is Your Relationship Universe.

Waldinger and Schulz suggest that you locate those people or groups that you would like to move from one quadrant to another. For example, I would like to move one of my friends into the upper right corner, which means I will need to create more opportunities to interact with him. Or say you want to move someone from the upper left to the upper right by creating more positive interactions with them. In my case, I often work out at a gym near my home, and one of the guys who I bump into there was getting

> under my skin. Well, I *let* him get under my skin. So, I first moved him to the lower left by working out at times he was unlikely to be at the gym. Now, I want to see if I can shift him to the upper right by finding ways to interact with him more positively. I will start by saying "Hello" instead of just putting my head down and ignoring him. We shall see, but at least I am going to try to be a relationship builder.

Let's now explore the characteristics of good relationships, whether they are simple and brief, or multifaceted and long lasting.

Being Known

At its most basic, being known arises from feeling that you are seen as a human being. It is lacking, for example, when someone is looking at their phone and fails to even acknowledge the person who is serving them at a store or restaurant. At a slightly deeper level, being known means that other people know your name and other basic information about you, the kind you share with a new acquaintance. At an even deeper level, being known occurs when two or more people have a sense of shared reality, a sense they see the world in the same way. This happens, for example, when you have the same opinion about an important topic or love the same sports team. Being known, of course, can grow deeper still with friends, families, and intimate partners.[8]

Being known grows when someone knows more about your core characteristics, the kind we will explore in chapter seven on authentic practices. This is the level of knowing that helps new friendships grow stronger. Sharing personal thoughts, feelings, and dreams is the deeper knowing among best friends, close family members, and intimate partners. Its basic principle: The more relationship partners know about each other, the deeper their experience of being known, and the stronger their relationship can grow.

Being Respected

At its most basic, being respected means feeling that your innate dignity as a person is being honored.[9] It rests on a nearly universal claim that all human beings have inherent and inalienable worth, which others must recognize and affirm. We feel respected, for example, when we feel appreciated by another person, they show positive regard for us, or they treat us courteously.

When we are treated disrespectfully, we may feel that our innate worth as a human has been disregarded, threatened, or impugned. This can happen when we are subject to even mild disrespect like being ignored or overlooked, or when we feel that our behavior has been misinterpreted or our motives misperceived. Consider a simple and all-too-common example: road rage. People can feel disrespected when a person they don't know and will likely never meet is tailgating them or cuts them off in traffic. In even the briefest encounters, people need to feel their value as a human being is recognized and honored.

Being Safe

Relationships can be risky. If someone gets to know us, then shows they do not like us, it hurts. Again, even brief encounters can feel threatening or safe. For a relationship to continue and grow, both parties need to feel psychologically safe to risk revealing more about themselves.[10] When safety is high, both people believe they can be authentic, who they really are, without fear of negative consequences. People who feel safe can express themselves honestly and appropriately in the relationship. Safety is essential for having productive disagreements instead of acrimonious arguments. When safety is low, people hold back important parts of themselves and refrain from investing in the relationship.

As you feel more fully known and respected, your sense of safety grows. You feel more secure in the relationship and more confident the other person will treat you well. Over time, relationship partners create what researchers call a safe haven: They can count on each other for support and protection when they feel uneasy, overwhelmed, or distressed. Research shows that feeling psychologically safe leads to a host of positive outcomes, including investing more in the relationship, better communication between relationship partners, greater freedom to be your best self, a greater capacity to learn new things, and strong support to grow and develop.

Being Valued

Scientists generally agree that all humans have a fundamental need to feel that other people like and value them.[11] Feeling valued is the glue that forms relational bonds between people; the stronger the valuing, the stronger the relational bonds. When we feel valued by another person, we believe they care about our welfare and want the best for us.[12] We experience valuing, for example, when someone does something positive to show they care about us—even simple acts of kindness. It matters in transitory relationships too: A genuine word of thanks to the person serving you at a store conveys you value them. At higher levels, we feel valued when someone expresses affection for us or takes care of us. The more valued we feel by another person, the more we know we can lean on them during difficult times.

Love, of course, is the fullest and richest expression of valuing another person. As social psychologist Barbara Fredrickson writes:

> Love, as it turns out, nourishes your body the way the right balance of sunlight, nutrient-rich soil, and water nourishes plants and allows them to flourish. The more you experience it, the more you open up and grow, becoming wiser and more attuned, more resilient and effective, happier and healthier. You grow spiritually as well, better able to see, feel, and appreciate the deep interconnections that inexplicably tie you to others, that embed you within the grand fabric of life.[13]

Being Supported

Being supported is being cared for by another person or persons. We can support others by providing helpful information, like answering a simple question, offering constructive feedback, or giving personal advice and counsel. We can support them by providing the things or assistance they need, like loaning someone a pen, carrying someone's luggage, making a meal for a friend, covering someone's living expenses while they look for a new job, or caring for someone while they are ill. And we can support them by providing emotional sustenance, like offering someone a simple thanks, telling a joke to lighten a coworker's mood, reassuring a friend who is feeling down, or cuddling a child.

The key insight from research is that high-quality relationships of all kinds—from one-time, transitory interactions to lifelong relationships, from those with one person to those with groups—are determined by the Play-Doh ball of these five elements. The amount of each of these relational characteristics—the size of the Play-Doh ball—varies across relationships. It's smaller for one-time interactions and much bigger for friends, family, and intimate partners. Nevertheless, to create positive connections, all of the elements must be present.

How to Be a Relationship Builder

How, then, can you build good relationships? As you are likely aware, there are dozens of books and resources on how to create and sustain intimate relationships, and I have listed some of the best in the Further Reading section. Here, we will cover the basic principles that apply to building and sustaining all kinds of relationships: availability, warmth, and responsiveness.[14] Let's take a look at each one.

Availability

It's hard to imagine forming any kind of relationship when the parties are completely absent from each other. Sure, even intimate couples can sustain strong relationships when they are physically apart for long periods, but the most basic and important form of availability is being present with each other, either in person or through another communication channel. It involves focusing your attention on another person with a benevolent orientation. You are paying attention to them with an attitude of goodwill, compassion, and kindness. Simply standing or sitting close to another person with this attitude can convey they are known, respected, safe, and valued.[15]

Imagine a conversation between two friends, Susanna and Jorge. Susanna shares a difficult experience she had with a coworker. While listening to her, Jorge maintains direct eye contact, nods affirmatively, asks helpful follow-up questions, and paraphrases specific details back to Susanna to ensure he understands. Now imagine a different scenario where Jorge frequently glances at his phone, occasionally mutters comments like "Uh-huh" and "Got it," and at one point abruptly changes the topic of conversation to his upcoming vacation. While he is physically present in both situations, Jorge is much more available in the first scenario.

One way to enhance your capacity to be more fully available is to practice empathy. Empathy is being sensitive to someone's emotional experiences. It is the capacity to place yourself in the "emotional shoes" of another person. One wise way to increase your capacity for empathy is by reading or watching fictional accounts of people's lives.[16]

PRACTICING EMPATHY

Reading fiction, watching emotionally compelling movies, and attending live theater offer opportunities to hone your skill at being empathic. When engaging in these kinds of activities, you can become immersed in the lives of the people and world presented to you. Fictional accounts create believable worlds that can become realistic to the reader or observer. People don't evaluate a good novel or movie for its consistency with reality but on whether it establishes a truth-likeness to real-life situations, which can draw you into the world of the fictional work. When you absorb a fictional story, you can find yourself identifying with its characters and becoming emotionally involved with their experiences, which, research suggests, enhances your capacity for empathy. The key is to allow yourself to be transported into the world of the story.[17]

Listening is another way to express availability. Becoming a good listener starts with a firm and positive intention to develop that capacity. Having a positive intention, as Haifa University researcher Guy Itzchakov and his colleagues write, "does not necessarily entail agreeing with the speaker or liking what they say. Instead, it involves conveying that one values, respects, and cares for the speaker *regardless* of what is said and a desire to understand the speaker's point of view to learn more about them."[18] High-quality listening creates a safe space so the other person feels comfortable sharing. As the first scenario with Susanna and Jorge illustrates, it involves paying attention to what someone is saying by maintaining eye contact, perhaps nodding your head affirmatively, and offering reassuring comments that convey your focus is on that person. Several wise practices can enhance your capacity to be a good listener. One ancient practice you can use with one person or a group is the Listening Circle.[19]

CREATE A LISTENING CIRCLE

A Listening Circle is a structured process for bringing people together to better understand one another while building and strengthening connection. Listening Circles have three features. First, every person must speak about something relevant to the conversation in the circle. Second, all circle members must listen with respectful attention. For example, any speaker must be allowed to fully offer what they want to say before another person begins to speak. This can be facilitated by passing a "talking stick" or other object around to ensure only the person holding it is speaking. Third, all circle participants must pay attention to the wellbeing of the circle. For example, each person must be aware of the impact of their contributions, both as a speaker and a listener, on the other participants. This includes, minimally, not judging or commenting on what other people share.

Kim and I have a similar practice we call "A Weather Report," for when we want to share something and would like the other person to simply listen and receive. The reporter has ten minutes to share what they wish. The receiver listens without offering any commentary. The report must end at ten minutes. This keeps us from circling around the problem again and again. If the reporter wants a response from the listener, they ask for it. The report always ends with an expression of affection, like a warm hug.

Availability is a powerful way to affirm another person is known, respected, and safe in your presence. It can be a part of everyday interactions when, for example, a partner responds in a timely manner to a text, coworkers eat lunch together, or you offer a brief but genuine greeting to someone you pass in a hallway or grocery aisle.

Warmth

A second key to being a relationship builder is offering genuine expressions of warmth such as acts of kindness, compassion, benevolence, generosity, and fun or playfulness. Warmth creates positive emotions that draw people together. When we express warmth toward another person we are signaling, "I see you, I respect you, I value you."

Genuine expressions of warmth are essential. We are highly sensitive to fraudulent expressions; most of us can easily sniff out when someone is pretending to be kind or generous. But even small and genuine gestures can convey warmth: a nice smile, a kind word, a text with a heart emoji, a sincere thanks. A wise practice for expressing warmth is what University of California, Santa Barbara, psychologist Shelly Gable calls capitalizing.

CAPITALIZING[20]

Positive things happen to most of us every day. Some are smaller events like finishing a work project, finding your favorite fresh berries at the grocery store, or hearing something funny from a child you know. Others are big like getting a new job you wanted, having a great first date with someone you like, or having your book proposal accepted by a fantastic publisher. Studies show that sharing these positive experiences has several benefits: boosting happiness, soothing distress, and strengthening bonds in new and existing relationships. These benefits are strongest when the receiving partner, the person hearing the good news, practices capitalization by responding actively and positively.

An active-positive response is one where you express interest and eagerness to hear the news, along with happiness, excitement, enthusiasm, pride, or another appropriate positive response. Genuineness is essential; you have to mean what you say. Responding actively and positively can also be accomplished by asking questions about the event. You might elaborate on the positive implications and benefits of the event or comment on why you think it is meaningful or important.

Active-positive responses work in several ways. They help maximize an event's value and memorability for your partner, they validate and amplify the value of the event itself, and they also signify that you value the person who shared the event. This makes experiences more memorable because the act of sharing entails reliving and elaborating on what happened, which increases its salience in memory. This creates a stronger and longer afterglow—the benefits of good experiences last longer than the events themselves.

Research also shows that most of us don't share our positive experiences very often. So, you might create a regular sharing practice with someone important to you. Kim and I often gather at the end of our work day to drink a glass of wine and share about our day. We are intentional about sharing at least one good thing from the day, no matter how difficult or trying it has been. When we talk to or get together with family members, we are also intentional about asking what is good in their lives and sharing back something that is good in ours. Positive sharing and capitalization practices do not take very much time, and even a few minutes can reap huge benefits.

In appropriate situations, another great way to express warmth is affectionate touch.[21] A hand on someone's shoulder, a light touch on their forearm, holding their hand, and other nonsexual touches can convey empathy, compassion, and kindness. When appropriate, hugging, kissing, and holding someone are even more powerful ways to communicate warmth. Touch can dial down a person's stress response, facilitate positive coping responses, and make them feel safe. Touch also can encourage positive sharing and cause the release of oxytocin, the so-called love hormone. Studies show that appropriate affectionate touch is one of the best ways to resolve conflict between partners.[22]

Responsiveness

Responsiveness describes how partners attend to and support each other's needs and goals.[23] Responsive relationship builders are proactive in reaching out to other people. They express warmth and sensitivity to their partners' feelings and actively engage in behaviors that make them feel known, safe, valued, and supported. When researchers ask people what they want from close relationships, they say things like having someone to confide in, to share life's joys with, and who can provide the support they need when they need it. Even when asked about interacting with transitory others like restaurant waitstaff or store sales associates, respondents say they seek positive behaviors, such as respectfulness, kindness, and cheerfulness. Receiving and providing responsiveness is good for everyone in the relationship, no matter how temporary.[24]

Researchers have found that in ongoing relationships, a wise form of responsiveness is engaging in practices that foster bringing out the best in our partners. The Michelangelo Practice is a wise way to help another person be at their best.[25]

THE MICHELANGELO PRACTICE

The great Renaissance artist Michelangelo Buonarroti reportedly described sculpting as releasing the ideal figure from the block of stone in which it slumbers. His task as a sculptor, he said, was to simply chip away at the stone to reveal the beautiful sculpture inherent in the marble. In relationships we, like this great artist, can imagine the best about our partners and act in ways that both reveal their best selves and help them develop and display those qualities.

To begin a Michelangelo Practice with a partner, spend time thinking about some of the things that make them special, what talents and strengths they possess, and the personality characteristics that make them uniquely wonderful. The more specific we can be about a partner's best-self qualities, the stronger will be the Michelangelo benefits. For example, saying "You work hard at learning new things and persist in learning even when at first it seems difficult" is more specific than saying "You're smart." I find that making a list of these things really helps me see the details I need to be able to offer better support. Like Michelangelo, the best sculptors "chip away," meaning they engage in a number of small behaviors that, over time, highlight and reinforce their partner's best self. Things like leaving affirming notes, capitalizing on their good news, and listening attentively are often the best kinds of sculpting. And remember, being genuine about your support is essential; we need to really believe what we are saying to our partners.

In a series of studies with intimate couples and friends, researchers found that when people received this kind of Michelangelo support, they actually developed, over time, more closely to their ideal self. In other words, positive sculpting from a partner helped them grow in self-integrity and authenticity.

In a lovely and very candid article, Northwestern University psychologist Eli Finkel recounts his initial disbelief in this phenomenon and how, through research and scholarly exploration, he came to develop a firm belief that it really works.[26] He uses the Michelangelo Practice as an entrée into research that shows how the metaphors we use to think about things powerfully affect the way we behave. This is especially true for the metaphors we use with relationships. If, for example, we think arguments are "a battle to see who is right," we are likely to engage in behaviors that attack our opponent's views. How might we respond if we used the metaphor that arguments are a dance between partners who are seeking a harmonious rhythm? He explores metaphors about love we might use: "I'm crazy about her" might suggest love is a kind of mental health challenge, or "He's magnetic" might suggest love is mostly a physical act. Finkel shares how adopting the metaphor that "love is a collaborative work" helped him become more responsive in the important relationships in his life. This article motivated me to be more intentional about surfacing the implicit metaphors that shape how I think about relationships in my life: partner to Kim, father, grandfather, work colleague, friend, and more. I am working to intentionally choose the metaphors that I want to shape how I interact with others.

Responsiveness enhances your capacity to understand your partner and, consequently, makes you a better responder. You become more aware of what your partner needs and more adept at providing it. For example, in a series of studies, researchers explored the factors that led first-year college roommates, who did not previously know each other, to form strong friendships.[27] As the students engaged in responsive behaviors like trying to make their roommate feel comfortable about themselves, being sensitive to their feelings, and listening to them when they talked, perceptions of respect, trust, and understanding grew. These friendships grew bit by bit through small acts of responsiveness. Another positive outcome of these responsive interactions is that they boosted both roommates' sense of self-integrity. In other words, having a responsive roommate made students feel better about themselves.

Sharing more about yourself is another wise way to be responsive.[28] Self-disclosures like sharing about the good things in your life and, in appropriate ways, the challenges you are facing are powerful relationship catalysts. Studies show, for example, that keeping a secret from a valued relationship partner tends to strain the relationship and undermine its quality, but confiding appropriately in them builds trust.[29] Arthur Aron, a legendary relationship researcher, developed a practice called Fast Friends that is highly effective in building new relationships and strengthening existing ones through mutual sharing.[30]

BECOMING FAST FRIENDS

Aron developed a set of thirty-six prompts that consecutively foster deeper sharing between partners. These prompts start by encouraging more modest sharing, providing answers to questions like "Given the choice of anyone in the world, whom would you want as a dinner guest?" "Would you like to be famous? If so, in what way? If not, why?" and "Before making a telephone call, do you ever rehearse what you are going to say? Why?" The prompts encourage deeper sharing, moving on to ones like "If a crystal ball could tell you the truth about yourself, your life, the future, or anything else, what would you want to know?" "Is there something that you've dreamed of doing for a long time? Why haven't you done it?" and "What is the greatest accomplishment of your life?" and ending with more intimate prompts like "Of all the people in your family, whose death would you find most disturbing? Why?" and "Share a personal problem and ask your partner's advice on how they might handle it. Ask your partner to reflect back to you how you seem to be feeling about the problem you have chosen." You can find the entire list at the Greater Good in Action website at ggia.berkeley.edu/practice/36_questions_for_increasing_closeness.

At some point in time, we all fall short in our availability, warmth, and responsiveness. "To err is human," Alexander Pope wrote, but research shows that forgiving is also very human and a powerful way to be responsive and overcome relationship failures or restore relationships after conflict.[31]

FORGIVENESS

Everett Worthington is probably the world's leading expert on forgiveness. He offers a variety of very useful exercises on his website (www.evworthington-forgiveness.com) for enhancing your capacity to practice it. These practices support his REACH model of forgiveness, which follows five steps:

First, *Recall* the hurt. Radical acceptance is important here. You have to face the fact that someone has hurt you significantly. Practice radical acceptance and acknowledge the injury, then form a clear intention to forgive the other person. Make a decision not to treat the other person as the villain.

Second, *Empathize* with the other person. For example, pretend they are in an empty chair across from you. Talk to them. Pour your heart out about the hurt you have experienced. Then, speak from that person's chair: Tell a human story of why you (remember, you are speaking as the other person) engaged in the hurtful action.

Third, offer the *Altruistic* gift of forgiveness. You might begin by remembering a time when you wronged someone else and that person forgave you. Remember how it felt to be forgiven. Then, form a clear intention to offer the gift of forgiveness to the person who hurt you. Forgiveness does not mean you condone or excuse their actions, but rather that you release them from the burden of their behavior and are no longer harboring ill feelings toward them.

Fourth, *Commit* to enacting that forgiveness. Act in concrete ways that show you are offering it to the other person. Sincerity is essential here, so be sure you are genuine in your gifts of forgiveness.

> Last, *Hold* on to forgiveness. It is entirely normal for your desire to forgive to wax and wane, so commit to continuing to forgive even when you doubt whether it is the right thing to do.

The key insight for nurturing connectedness is to be a relationship builder. Someone in the relationship has to make the first responsive, warm, supportive gesture. When that gesture is reciprocated, it creates a positive, upward spiral through which mutual respect, trust, and care deepen and grow. Yale University professor and relationship expert Margaret Clark writes, "We need to know that we are not needlessly expending our energy and time, foolishly building our hopes, and dangerously feeling attached and revealing vulnerabilities to people who will hurt us. In short, we need to be confident that partners want what we want . . . Were it not for [responsiveness], relationship partners might often arrive at an interdependence stalemate, neither making a move until he or she is sure of the other's intentions."[32] There are wise ways to express availability, warmth, and responsiveness in many different contexts, even in ones like work, where interactions may tend to be transactional instead of relational. University of Pennsylvania organizational psychologist Adam Grant, whom we met in chapter four, has been a leading researcher and advocate for prosocial relationships at work. He characterizes this as being a giver instead of a taker, describing the difference this way:

> Whereas takers tend to be self-focused, evaluating what other people can offer them, givers are other-focused, paying more attention to what other people need from them . . . Givers and takers differ in their attitudes and actions toward other people.

> If you're a taker, you help others strategically, when the benefits to you outweigh the personal costs. If you're a giver, you might use a different cost-benefit analysis: you help whenever the benefits to others exceed the personal costs. Alternatively, you might not think about the personal costs at all, helping others without expecting anything in return. If you're a giver at work, you simply strive to be generous in sharing your time, energy, knowledge, skills, ideas, and connections with other people who can benefit from them.[33]

Of course, sometimes takers will take advantage of your giving, so there are limits to it. But Grant's research shows that more often than not, giving is good for both givers and receivers. And generosity, kindness, and goodwill spread. If you lead with giving to build strong relationships at work or in other social settings, you will likely be a catalyst for others to give as well.

KEY INSIGHTS

Strong, mutually supportive social relationships in all areas of our life are essential for our wellbeing. We need to feel known, respected, safe, valued, and supported even in life's temporary interactions, and we need to offer those kinds of relationships to the people we interact with.

The key is to be a relationship builder. Use simple practices like the ones in this chapter to create and strengthen high-quality relationships. To build good relationships, focus on being present and available, creating warmth and acceptance, and proactively responding to partners' needs.

Reaching greater depths of self-disclosure between partners is the key to building greater trust.

Forgiveness is among the wisest practices for restoring relationships.

FURTHER READING

The Emotional Lives of Teenagers: Raising Connected, Capable, and Compassionate Adolescents by Lisa Damour: Insightful and packed with authoritative advice. I wish I had this book when my boys were teenagers.

The All-or-Nothing Marriage: How the Best Marriages Work by Eli J. Finkel: One of the best evidence-based books about creating and sustaining intimate relationships.

The Science of Trust: Emotional Attunement for Couples by John M. Gottman: A deep dive into the science of trust by one of its leading researchers. Helpful for building trust in all kinds of relationships.

Give and Take: Why Helping Others Drives Our Success by Adam Grant: A skillful exploration of how generosity, kindness, and putting other people first can be good for others and for yourself.

Hold Me Tight: Seven Conversations for a Lifetime of Love by Sue Johnson: While this book focuses primarily on intimate relationships, the insights and advice are also helpful for building strong connections with friends and family.

Social Chemistry: Decoding the Patterns of Human Connection by Marissa King: A great exploration of networking and how to use it effectively.

CHAPTER SEVEN

Authentic Practices

Building Self-Integrity

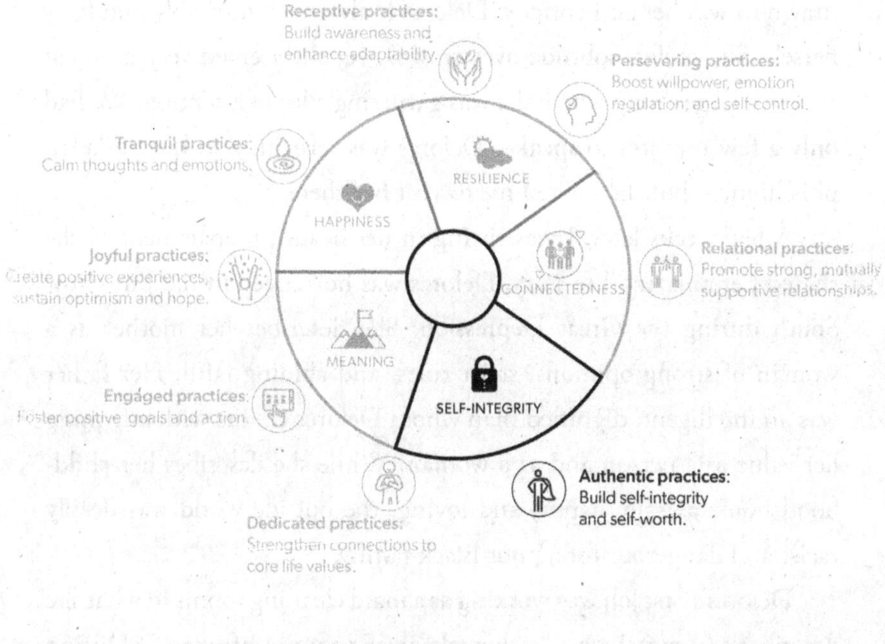

The day I first met Delores Flynn Brisbon, I had just finished the keynote speech at a conference of two thousand senior leaders of religious organizations. On days like that, I am eager to retreat to the nearest park to walk off the post-speech stress. On this day, however, a colleague found me and said Delores wanted to meet me. I knew she was an accomplished and highly respected leader. He encouraged me that this was an opportunity I should embrace. I wanted to demur, but his encouragement—"Delores is an amazing and wise person. You will be glad you met her!"—compelled me to go with him.

As I approached her table, she called out my name and "insisted" I sit next to her. It was the kind of insistence that was mirthful and inviting. Delores, a dignified and cultivated woman in her late eighties, was warm, kind, and generous to me, as she is to everyone. What I felt most drawn to was her authenticity. Delores is always comfortably and fully herself. She prefers solitude over crowds, yet she seemed very much at ease in a large group where she was garnering a lot of attention. We had only a few minutes to speak—Delores was returning to her Philadelphia home—but she invited me to visit her there.

A few weeks later, I was sitting in her beautiful apartment as she shared her amazing life story. Delores was born deep in the Jim Crow South during the Great Depression. She describes her mother as a woman of strong opinions, strict rules, and abiding faith. Her father was an intelligent, dignified man whom Delores credits with affirming her value as a person and as a woman. While she describes her childhood home as safe, happy, and loving, the outside world was deeply racist and dangerous for a poor Black family.

Delores's first job was working as a maid cleaning rooms in what she describes as a motel with "a clientele given to unfaithfulness."[1] During that time, she applied to the Tuskegee Institute and was accepted to their school of nursing. After graduation she took a nursing position at a small local hospital. That was the beginning of her long, successful career in healthcare. Several years later, an aunt urged her to move to Philadelphia because of the good, higher-paying jobs for nurses at large hospitals there.

For a Black woman, however, Philadelphia was hardly the city of brotherly or sisterly love. Delores experienced hostility and racism in myriad forms. She was given the most difficult assignments; parts of her uniform would mysteriously disappear from her locker, replaced with hateful notes; and a more senior white nurse once told her that "the place for colored people is caring for our children." She even received threatening phone calls at her home. Nevertheless, Delores continued her exemplary work, which earned her the respect of senior leaders and a series of promotions. Her career culminated with her appointment as the chief operations officer at a large healthcare system.

Many experiences in Delores's life could have damaged her self-integrity. Nevertheless, throughout her career, coworkers described her as quietly confident and self-assured. One longtime colleague said the thing she admired most about Delores was her insistence on "the absolute necessity of knowing and valuing oneself." In her second autobiography, *A Privileged Life II*, Delores writes, "I have lived and celebrated the unique human being I am made to be, free and authentic."[2] She writes that throughout her life, family, community, church, and teachers

> gave me the wisdom to be myself . . . I am a shy, tall, black woman with curly hair, and a big smile, and a good listener with a compassionate heart. I prefer to engage in small groups,

> even individually, which eliminates a desire to be included in many activities common to others and not enjoyed by me. If my presence does not contribute to an outcome, small or large, I prefer not to be involved, not as judgment of others, but it is what fits who I know myself to be . . . We are not at risk when we know ourselves. As we change, mature, and make choices, our life is consistent. We act from the core of who we are, not from situations or circumstances.[3]

Delores is firm in her conviction that "being myself has been at the root of every natural achievement personally, professionally, and socially." It was the source of strength she needed to navigate racism and life tragedies, and to excel in difficult and demanding circumstances. In this chapter we will explore the science of how authentic practices can empower you to develop and sustain, like Delores, a strong sense of self-integrity.

The Autobiographical Roots of Self-Integrity

In chapter two I described self-integrity as having a balanced, secure, and overall positive identity. It is seeing yourself as a good, capable, moral person who is striving to live a good life and make important contributions to other people and the world around you. All of the things you hold to be true about who you are form your identity.

To understand how wise practices can strengthen and sustain self-integrity, we will explore insights from Life Narrative Theory, one of the most illuminating scientific explanations of how our identity is formed. Throughout history, the theory asserts, humans have relied on stories to understand the important things in their lives, such as how the world works, what it means to live a good life, and being human. Through myths, legends, novels, songs, and more, we tell and hear stories that help us navigate the complexities of life. Pulitzer Prize–winning journalist Tomas Alex Tizon captures why stories are so important:

> Stories give shape to experience and allow us to go through life unblind. Without them, everything that happens would float around, undifferentiated. None of it would mean anything. Once you have a version of what happened, all the other good stuff about being human comes into play. You can laugh, feel awe, commit a passionate act, get pissed, want to change things.[4]

Psychologists have found that our identities—our sense of who we are and how we fit into the world—are formed through the process of mentally authoring the story of our lives, our life narrative. This process begins in adolescence when our brains develop the capacity to create complex stories.[5] Whether you realize it or not, every day since you were in your teens you have been authoring a mental story about yourself. It has chapters that cover important periods of your life, and is full of stories about the significant people and important events that have shaped you. It includes descriptions and details of how you have changed, for better and sometimes for worse.

You can test this for yourself. Consider three memories: your senior year in high school, what your day was like last Saturday, and your most recent trip to a store. If you recall those memories, each of them will be a mental story. Even something as everyday and simple as going to a store is, at least for a time, a story in your life narrative.

Important periods in your life, like your senior year in high school, are collections of stories linked together to tell the grand narrative of an important time.

Your life narrative is the entire collection of memories, vignettes, chronicles, anecdotes, and reminiscences that are woven together to tell the story of you and how you became the person you are. It contains adventure stories, dramas, tragedies, comedies, and other kinds of stories, each one telling something important about you and your life.

Before this discovery, psychologists struggled to develop a cogent, comprehensive account of how we construct our identities. We don't walk around thinking of ourselves as just a bunch of facts and descriptors (I'm six feet tall; I was a professor; I am married to Kim). Let's face it, that would be immensely difficult because each of us is incredibly complicated. Even so, we experience ourselves as, well, ourselves—as a whole person that certainly has characteristics and qualities we can describe, but those descriptions don't fully capture who we really are or how we think about ourselves. It is by constructing a rich, detailed, exciting, sometimes bewildering but always evolving life story that we make all those descriptions come alive as the person we are.

If you could somehow print out your life story, it would require thousands of pages. Even so, you somehow carry all those pages in your mind, and you can access most chapters and stories with ease. Your life narrative is part autobiography: It contains your history and the past events, people, and experiences that are important parts of you. It includes chapters and stories about who you are today and what's happening in your life right now. And you are writing stories about who you might be and what might happen to you in the future, whether that is tomorrow or years from now. All of these elements create your sense of "who I really am."

Researchers call this understanding of "who I really am" authenticity.[6] It is the key to self-integrity: Authenticity arises from authoring a life story through which you understand and accept, if not celebrate, the unique human being you are. It is by gaining this kind of rich self-understanding that you are able to form a balanced, secure, and positive identity. In other words, authoring an authentic life story, one that tells who you really are and how you became that person, creates self-integrity.

Many of the self-help offerings that claim to improve self-worth and self-confidence can't work because they don't focus on life narratives. It's hard to directly change self-worth by trying to think better of yourself or focusing on the good things about you because those approaches focus on the facts of your story. They don't integrate positive self-understandings into the deeper story from which self-worth and self-confidence emerge. Let's explore what science tells us about how we create authenticity and how wise practices can strengthen yours.

Authoring an Authentic Life Narrative

Throughout this chapter I use verbs like "write," "craft," and "author" to describe the mental processes we use to create our life narrative, and I do this to convey several important insights. The first is that you are the main writer of your narrative. True, some of that writing has been done in your subconscious, and some of the stories and details are incomplete, but nevertheless you are the author. And that leads to the second insight: You can strengthen your self-integrity by being a more intentional author. You have a lot of editorial license to write and rewrite sections of your life story. This editorial capacity will be a key for authoring an authentic life narrative and creating a strong sense of self-integrity. As Delores reflected, her willingness to take responsibility to live and celebrate her uniqueness and character was essential for her capacity to affirm her authentic self.

A third insight is that other people influence your life story, sometimes in very helpful ways, like when they encourage you to embrace your good qualities, and sometimes in hurtful ways, like when they ostracize or malign you. The social cultures we live in at work, in our social groups, and in communities also shape our life story, again sometimes for the better (e.g., when social norms shifted to more fully honor women and nonheterosexuality) and sometimes for the worse (e.g., systemic racism that denies full personhood to people of color). Choose your coauthors carefully. Yes, it can be hard to withstand powerful social forces when they urge you to measure yourself against other people or when social structures devalue essential parts of who you are. Wise practices that help you enhance and sustain authenticity can be powerful ways to resist those pressures. Consider the social environment Delores grew up in that denied her personhood, and how important people in her life validated and affirmed her unique strengths, personality, and value. That social support was essential in her ability to craft her "free and authentic" identity.

A final insight is that authoring your life story is a lifelong endeavor. It will continue to expand, evolve, and change. You don't need to revise everything right away; you can take time to be a thoughtful and careful author. Taking a long-term perspective on your life story can create the psychological space and motivation to learn how to be more intentional about the ways you revise old chapters and write new ones.

Let's now explore what science tells us about how we can author an authentic life narrative by enhancing self-awareness, increasing core self-knowledge, and foregrounding (discovering, revealing, and describing) important parts of your life narrative.

Harness Self-Awareness

Authoring an authentic life narrative requires a certain capacity of self-awareness to perceive yourself candidly and comprehensively.[7] Here, self-awareness facilitates the exploration and acceptance of your inherent characteristics and qualities, what researchers call your core self. Self-awareness creates the self-discovery, as Delores writes, that leads to knowing and valuing yourself.

Writing about your life is one of the wisest ways of cultivating self-understanding. Keeping a diary or life journal is a time-tested, evidence-based practice. It is beneficial on its own, and (as we will see) it is also a building block for other authentic practices. Novelist and journal writer Susan Sontag deftly captured the benefits of this practice: "In the journal I do not just express myself more openly than I could do to any person; I create myself. The journal is a vehicle for my sense of selfhood."[8] Journaling regularly is a simple and powerful way to engage in reflection and introspective examination of yourself and your life.

JOURNALING

A handwritten journal is best because technology often creates obstacles to the free flow of thoughts that are key to making this practice effective. Research suggests that writing by hand has important advantages over typing or dictating.[9] It contributes extensively to the brain's connectivity patterns that promote learning and memory, whereas typing does not engage these neural growth processes. Another key to effective journaling is to be open and honest about what's going on in your daily life.

You can use a very simple journaling format, such as answering three questions each day: What are the main things that happened today? What do I think about those happenings? What do I feel about those happenings? Insights about why you think and feel arise best from first describing them, so first write about *what* you thought and felt. After several days (or even better, weeks), look back over your entries for patterns in your thoughts and feelings. You will see answers to *why* you thought and felt those ways in these descriptions.

Another format is to use the Map Your Days practice in chapter one, where you record a high and low point each day. You can adapt it by journaling about what you thought and felt about those highs and lows.

Keep it simple! A simple format will allow you to spend more time in introspection and self-reflection. Over time, you will become more skillful in being aware of your thoughts, feelings, and motives, and more skillful in understanding what lies underneath them.

Write at least several days a week about what is going on in your life right now. It's important to commit to journaling even when you don't think you have anything to write about. Each morning, I write three handwritten, stream-of-consciousness pages about my life. I have found that this three-page commitment, especially when I am at a loss about what to write, is a great way to push my thinking deeper into self-awareness. By the time I am on page two, if not earlier, thoughts and insights are emerging that wouldn't have if I had stopped at a paragraph or two. If you keep this commitment to journaling, you will almost certainly find that it unlocks important insights for you.

While self-discovery practices are important, the insights and feedback from trusted others can be helpful in developing the self-awareness that leads to authenticity. We all have coauthors, so selecting the right ones and collaborating more actively with them is a wise practice. The trick is to get candid feedback, the kind of information that others might be reluctant to share. Organizational psychologist Tasha Eurich recommends a wise practice called the Dinner of Truth.[10]

THE DINNER OF TRUTH

Choose someone who knows you well, such as a family member or close friend, and invite them to a meal. Explain that during the meal you will ask them to tell you one thing that annoys them the most about you. Tell them you're doing this because you want to increase self-awareness, and understanding the negative ways you show up with others is an important and necessary part of helping you grow. Explain that you will listen with an open heart and mind, and not respond until they are finished. Then you will only ask clarifying questions.

Spend some time anticipating what might be said. Prepare for the worst-case scenario and resolve to remain quiet and in control of your facial and bodily gestures. Be clear with yourself about how much you are willing to hear. If there are subjects you want to be off limits, tell your invited guest.

When the dinner is over, journal about what you heard. Try to record the person's feedback as accurately as you can. Then, take time to journal about what you can learn from it. Last, write some thoughts about how you might use this feedback to grow and change in positive ways.

Reflections and insights accumulate, and "aha!" moments of deeper self-understanding bubble up from this accumulation. Be patient and continue taking small steps. Scrutinize emerging insights. Your capacity for self-awareness will increase over time.

Some religious traditions offer spiritual disciplines that are designed to increase self-awareness. The Roman Catholic practice of the Daily Examen is one such practice, and it can be adapted for nonreligious use.

THE DAILY EXAMEN

The Daily Examen comprises five movements or phases:

1. Place yourself in God's presence. Give thanks for God's great love for you.
2. Pray for the grace to understand how God is acting in your life.
3. Review your day, recalling specific moments and feelings.

4. Reflect on what you did, said, or thought in those instances. Were you drawing closer to God, or farther away?
5. Look toward tomorrow—think of how you might collaborate more effectively with God's plan.

A secular version might follow these five movements:

1. Place yourself in a calm and peaceful state.
2. Express gratitude for the day that has just passed.
3. Review the high and low points of your day, recalling your thoughts, feelings, and actions.
4. Reflect on what you did, said, or thought. Where were these positive? Where were these negative?
5. Think of how you might live more positively in the day ahead.

Sometimes the process of increased self-awareness can bring up troubling thoughts and feelings. If this becomes burdensome, seek the guidance of a mental health professional. A trained therapist can help you deal effectively with the distress you might experience and also support you with helpful self-discovery and self-understanding.

Increase Knowledge of Your Core Characteristics

Harnessing self-awareness unlocks your capacity for discovering and describing the qualities, personality traits, passions, core values and beliefs, and other characteristics that are most emblematic of your truest, most authentic self. Each of us has hundreds of attributes, from the foods we like, to the talents we have, to our enduring dispositions and preferences. Many of those characteristics are not essential to your sense of yourself. I like Brussels sprouts, wear a size 11½ shoe, and have brown eyes, but those aren't part of my authentic self. Core characteristics define, for better and for worse, who you truly are.

The idea that each person has an authentic or true self has a long history going back to at least the ancient Greek aphorism "Know thyself." Aristotle, for example, taught that we all have a true self that we can discover through rigorous self-examination. The great psychologist William James claimed, "There is but one cause of human failure. And that is man's lack of faith in his true self."[11] Legendary psychologists including Carl Jung, Abraham Maslow, and Carl Rogers viewed the authentic self as a set of innate attributes each person is born with, and that full psychological functioning requires that we discover and accept these core characteristics.

An important insight from narrative identity research is that understanding and embracing your core characteristics is essential for building an authentic identity and maintaining self-integrity. There are always new things you can learn about yourself, but a good place to start is to identify some of your most important strengths, personality traits, and enduring preferences. (Knowing your core life values is also an essential part of authenticity, which we will explore in chapter eight on dedicated practices.)

Strengths are your important talents, skills, and positive capacities. Examples include being imaginative or courageous, having high emotional intelligence, being a good problem solver, having a strong musical talent, and being a natural leader. Some of mine are that I'm creative, a good teacher, and highly capable in emergency situations. Strengths form the basis for the kinds of activities and work you can perform well. Regularly using your strengths has other benefits such as boosting happiness and increasing resilience.[12] Remember, your strengths are what *you* can do well, not what you can do compared to what other people can do. I can be a good teacher without regard to whether other people are "better" teachers.

A study of organizational leaders by researchers at the University of Florida shows how reflecting on strengths can boost wellbeing.[13] They started with the premise that being a leader can be demanding and energy depleting, so maintaining good leadership can be a challenge. They hypothesized that by reflecting on their strengths, leaders could maintain or even restore the energy they need for work. Each morning for ten days, half of the leaders engaged in a series of simple reflections on their strengths; for example, they wrote about "three things you like about yourself that make you a good leader" or "three valuable skills you have that make you a good leader." Participants in the control group wrote each morning about a normal experience they had as a leader. At the end of each day everyone was asked to report how much energy they had during the day and how depleted they felt at day's end. These researchers were especially clever because they made sure every leader was in both the strengths-reflection group and control group for a period of time. On days when leaders spent time reflecting on strengths, they reported significantly greater energy at work and lower daily depletion. They were also more self-confident and felt they were more effective as a leader on those days.

Personality traits are like your basic operating system, forming the enduring patterns of the ways you think, feel, and act. When we describe someone as an introvert or extrovert, we are usually characterizing their overall "style" as a person. Your personality traits form your distinctive way of experiencing and interacting with other people and the world around you. If you are highly conscientious, for example, then you tend to be very responsible and hardworking; you place high value on honoring the commitments you have made to others. If you are highly open, you tend to be curious and imaginative. You value learning and exploring new things.

The "Five-Factor Model" is the most widely researched taxonomy of personality traits. You can remember the factors using the mnemonic OCEAN:

- Openness to experience (how open minded, imaginative, creative, and insightful a person is)
- Conscientiousness (how efficient, organized, and responsible a person is)
- Extroversion (how outgoing, energetic, and sociable a person is)
- Agreeableness (how friendly, compassionate, and kind a person is)
- Neuroticism (how anxious, nervous, and emotionally unstable a person is)

More recently, some researchers have proposed a sixth trait, honesty and humility (how trustworthy, modest, and sincere a person is). The Open-Source Psychometric Project (openpsychometrics.org/tests/IPIP-BFFM/) offers a free online version of an excellent assessment.

Personality traits create relatively stable patterns that are not locked in or prescriptive. Even introverts sometimes respond in more extroverted ways, and even the most conscientious person can occasionally be forgetful or capricious. Research also shows that our personality can change.[14] Furthermore, studies suggest that one of the ways getting older can also be getting better is that our personalities tend to change for the better. A study of more than 100,000 adults found that older adults were more conscientious and agreeable and less emotionally reactive than younger adults.[15]

Enduring preferences are the strong, consistent interests and passions that are essential parts of you. Enduring interests come in myriad forms, but they are different from things that are fun to do or that you enjoy. They shape the kinds of activities you love to do, the ones you are passionate about. If you could not participate in them, your life would be diminished. And you identify with them. For example, I love learning, I'm a bookworm, and I'm an avid scuba diver. Notice that last statement: I claimed scuba diving as part of my identity. It's not just something I do; it's part of who I am. I know someone who is passionate about model trains, spending a lot of time working on elaborate train models and learning about train history. Some of his closest friendships are with other model railroaders.

Strengths, personality traits, and enduring preferences form some of the core characteristics that make you, you. As I have mentioned, other parts of yourself are also integral to your authentic self. People who know you well can be immensely helpful in discovering these core characteristics. I have used this next wise practice with hundreds of graduate students and working professionals. Although some were reluctant at first to try it, people always praised the experience as one of the most helpful for learning important things about themselves.

REFLECTED BEST-SELF STORIES

Significant people in our lives like family, friends, teachers, pastors, coaches, and bosses can provide insights about our core self-characteristics by sharing what they know about us. This practice involves selecting five or six of these significant people from different parts of your life. Limit yourself to one family member so you can gain the insights of a diverse group. Ask each person to write about a time they saw you at your best. Ask them to write about what happened, the other people involved, and, most importantly, what you did during that episode. Then, have them summarize what you can learn from what they shared. You might be hesitant to ask, but people are usually honored to be invited to help you.[16]

After you have received all these stories, write your own summary of what you learned. Begin with a statement like, "At my best I . . ." and then write! Don't censor yourself. Be generous with your description. Remember, you are not comparing yourself to other people, you are working to gain personal insights. If you wish, you can share this description with some of your writers, or with other significant people, and invite them to reflect with you.

At some point you will need to turn your attention to the negative elements of your core self. Carl Jung called this our shadow self, "the thing [a person] has no wish to be."[17] Its elements include persistent biases and prejudices; strong desires like a lust for power; and stubborn, problematic tendencies like perfectionism or procrastination. We often dislike these shadow characteristics, but exploring and surfacing them allows us to deal effectively with them. One of mine is that a part of me wants to be famous. At this point in my life, I am sure that fame would be unrewarding and potentially detrimental, but there was a time when I worked hard to achieve it. Acknowledging that persistent desire allowed me to understand and deal with it so that, over time, it has diminished considerably. I still have to be mindful of the impulse to seek fame, and thankfully I have developed wise practices that help me manage it well.

Clinical psychologist Rick Hanson, an expert on self-discovery, says that 80 percent of what we learn about ourselves will be good things.[18] Even so, sometimes exploring and learning about your core self can be troubling. Again, consulting a mental health expert can be very helpful if you run into difficulties.

Another tool for mitigating some of the negative thoughts and feelings that might emerge from self-discovery is practicing self-compassion. University of Texas psychologist Kristin Neff, who conducted groundbreaking research on self-compassion, describes it as being supportive toward yourself when you experience suffering or pain caused by personal mistakes, your shadow self, or external life challenges.[19] Self-compassion has three elements: practicing radical acceptance, displaying self-kindness, and embracing your common humanity.

In self-compassion, radical acceptance comes from acknowledging and affirming the pain and suffering you are experiencing. It means truly accepting your inner experiences of injury, heartache, or distress. Self-kindness involves more than ending self-criticism; it is actively showing yourself the same kind of care and concern you would a suffering loved one. Embracing common humanity is recognizing that life challenges are part of being human. As Professor Neff describes it, "Our struggles are what make us card-carrying members of humankind . . . It implies a basic mutuality in the experience of suffering, and it springs from the acknowledgment that the human experience is imperfect."[20]

SELF-COMPASSION

Begin this practice by recalling a time when you cared for and stood by another person. It might be a child you were caring for, a friend you were encouraging, or a parent facing difficult health issues. Allow yourself to remember that experience, especially how it felt to support that person. Recall where those feelings were in your body, including the expressions on your face as you actively cared for them. Also take a moment to remember some of your intentions. Create a vivid image of you caring for the other person.

Then take a moment to apply this attitude to yourself. Imagine being an ally to yourself, someone who will look out for you, help you, and protect you. Try to embrace the fact that you have needs that matter and you have a right to be cared for. If other reactions come up, such as feeling unworthy, step back so you can recognize that everyone has that need. Then go back to offering that care for yourself.

Another self-compassion practice is remembering a time when you were really on your own side. Perhaps you stood up for yourself when someone mistreated you, or you were proud of something you did. Take note of the feelings you experienced and where they were located in your body. Recall some of the thoughts you had. Stay with this experience and let it fill your mind. Know what it's like to care for your own wellbeing. Let the feelings, thoughts, and intentions of being a true friend to yourself sink in, becoming a part of you.

As you discover more of your core self-characteristics, you will be creating a big, rich, and complex "picture" of who you are, a storied self-portrait. Bit by bit you will be able to add new details, which will enhance that picture and enrich your understanding of yourself. A wise practice that can aid that understanding is to literally create a picture of you.

MAKE THE PICTURE OF YOU

Start with a large piece of paper, newsprint, or posterboard, one with plenty of room to draw finer details. Gather drawing tools; colored pencils are particularly helpful. Begin by drawing pictorial representations of your core self-characteristics. If knowledge and learning are important, you might draw a library and title the books with your areas of expertise and interest. If an athletic endeavor is an essential part of you, draw that activity in a way that represents why it is important and how you feel about it. You might sketch yourself high-fiving your teammates or practicing a drill that will improve your skill. Also, draw the social roles that are part of who you are, the relationships that are essential to you, and the important groups you belong to. Imagine ways to draw your personality. For example, if you are an introvert, you might draw a cozy room or cave and decorate it with symbols of why that characteristic is an authentic part of you. If you're an extrovert, you might draw a party with people engaging in conversations and activities that make you feel energized and alive. Take your time with this picture. Add elements and details over time. It might seem hard at first, but eventually ideas and images will more readily come to mind. Consider sharing your picture with some of the important people in your life; you might even invite them to add their ideas and drawings to it.

Another version of this practice is to gather pictures of yourself from various points in your life. Write a story about what you were like at the time of each picture. Describe some of your most prominent core self-characteristics, and then write a story about some of the things you did and experiences you had that illustrate how those characteristics showed up during that time in your life. A good way to end is to write a note of appreciation for the person in each picture and the important ways they shaped you to be the person you are today.

Foreground Your Life Stories

Given that your identity is "written" into a life story, be sure to foreground some of the significant stories of your life.[21] These include stories about the important chapters, events, and people that have shaped you; the key transition points in your life; and the ways you have changed and grown over time. Foregrounding is an active, intentional process of remembering important parts of your life story; recounting, chronicling, and describing those parts; and linking them together in a way similar to a good novel. It lets you be a more intentional author, and will help you gain a fuller, more holistic, clearer sense of who you are and how you became that person.

Without this capacity to foreground key elements of our life narrative, we would have to try to recreate ourselves every day. *The Bourne Identity*, a film about fictitious CIA operative Jason Bourne, illustrates how profound this loss would be. Bourne experiences a traumatic event that erases his capacity to craft his life narrative. He loses all of his memories of himself. As a result, he is unable to piece together who he is. In a conversation with a confidant, he says,

> I can tell you the license plate numbers of all six cars outside. I can tell you that our waitress is left-handed and the guy sitting up at the counter weighs two hundred fifteen pounds and knows how to handle himself. I know the best place to look for a gun is the cab of the gray truck outside, and at this altitude, I can run flat out for a half mile before my hands start shaking. Now why would I know that? How can I know that and not know who I am?

Although, thankfully, most of us have not experienced this kind of extreme loss, we may still have gaps in our understanding of who we are and how we became that person. Foregrounding stories from important periods of life and actually writing about them is a simple and very wise practice that can yield huge benefits.

WRITE ABOUT IMPORTANT CHAPTERS FROM YOUR LIFE

We return here to the foundational practice of journaling, but adapt it to foreground important parts of your life story. Northwestern University psychologist Dan McAdams is an expert on Life Narrative Theory, and his Life Story Interview (tiny.cc/LifeNarrative) is a great tool to guide you in this journaling practice. McAdams has established the effectiveness of this tool in studies with hundreds of people. You can use it as a guide for writing about important parts of your life story.

Begin by imagining that your life story is a book with a table of contents that lists the main chapters of your life. Each chapter covers an important period in your life. Write a title for each chapter and a brief, one-paragraph summary of what it is about. This creates the overall plot line of your life story. Remember you can, and likely will, change any of this any time you wish. You may add new chapters, take out some, change the titles, rewrite the summaries. All of that editing is part of learning more about who you are and how you became that person.

After you have created this table of contents, a good place to turn is to write about a high point in your life, which McAdams describes this way:

> *Please describe a scene, episode, or moment in your life that stands out as an especially positive experience. This might be* the *high-point scene of your entire life, or else an especially happy, joyous, exciting, or wonderful moment in*

the story. Please describe this high-point scene in detail. What happened, when and where, who was involved, and what were you thinking and feeling? Also, please say a word or two about why you think this particular moment was so good and what the scene may say about who you are as a person.[22]

Just put words down without censoring or wordsmithing what you write. You are not trying to write a literary masterpiece; you are doing this for yourself.

Next, write about a low point that stands out as an especially difficult or challenging period in your life. You've likely had several high and low points, so write about several of each.

From there, you can explore other key moments in your life like positive and negative memories from childhood that shaped your early sense of yourself, vivid memories of events that had a profound impact on you, mastery and failure experiences where you learned about the skills and capabilities you have and those you don't, turning points in which your life changed in significant ways, and times you acted especially wisely or admirably.

As you make progress, pause from time to time to write a description of the main character, the "you" that is emerging in those stories. Write from a third-person point of view, as if you are describing the main character for a book.

I have used this tool in my research to gather life stories from hundreds of people. With very few exceptions, they said it was one of the best experiences they have ever had. Many told me it was a life-changing experience because they learned important things about themselves and came away with a stronger understanding of who they are.

As you become a more intentional author, you can rewrite stories in ways that turn them into positive parts of your life narrative. When you foreground a painful story from your past, for example, you can rewrite it as a time you discovered something important about yourself, other people, or the world around you. You can turn memories of personal failures into stories of personal growth. Or, you can write about the silver linings in stories about life crises.

In his memoir *Dreams from My Father*, future President Barack Obama recounts key events from his past as he describes growing from being a confused young adult struggling to find himself, into an adult who had a clear sense of meaning and purpose.[23] His African father abandoned him and his mother when he was a baby. Raised initially in rural Kansas, he learned to "slip back and forth between my black and white worlds," hoping to somehow connect the two.[24] The moves his family made to Hawaii, then Indonesia, then back to Hawaii taught him that race shapes people's perceptions. His years in New York during and after college were a pivotal period of self-discovery, in which

> a whole bunch of stuff that had been inside me—questions of identity, questions of purpose, questions of, not just race, but also the international nature of my upbringing—all those things [were] converging in some way. And so there's this period of time when I move to New York and go to Columbia where I pull in and wrestle with that stuff, and do a lot of writing and a lot of reading and a lot of thinking and a lot of walking through Central Park. And somehow I emerge on the other side of that

ready and eager to take a chance in what is a pretty unlikely venture: moving to Chicago and becoming an organizer.[25]

Over time, he learns that his "stories, taken together, helped me bind my world together," which gave him "the sense of place and purpose I'd been looking for."[26] Like President Obama's, our life stories are complex and complicated. It's unlikely we will ever be able to author a life narrative in which everything we know about ourselves fits neatly together. The good news from research is that to become more authentic, we don't need to craft a narrative that captures and neatly integrates all of the important details of our life. We just need enough richness and integration to feel like we know who we are and how we became that way.

Reading memoirs of those we admire can be very helpful for showing how to do this. As we learn about how these people were able to weave the many facets of their core self and the many significant experiences of their life together into a coherent-enough life narrative of their authentic self, we can gain insights into how we can do this as well.

READ MEMOIRS

Biographies and autobiographies tend to be descriptive. They tell important facts about a person's life. Memoirs reveal how the author views their life and how they came to understand their authentic self. Choose memoirs written by people you admire because the messiness and complexity of their narratives will likely resonate more with your own. Resist highlighting passages or making notes so you can let their full story unfold. Wait until you finish the book to write reflections on what you read. Try to map the plot line of their story, noting pivotal events and significant people and how these shaped the author's authentic sense of themself. Look for life themes that unfolded over time. Then, look for parallels with your life story, or insights you can apply to yours.

KEY INSIGHTS

Self-integrity—having a balanced, secure, and overall positive identity—arises from having an authentic sense of yourself; that is, from knowing the most essential characteristics that make you, you.

Understanding these essential characteristics involves exploring, identifying, and accepting your strengths, your personality, your passions and preferences, and your core values. It also involves acknowledging and accepting your shadow self.

Because your identity is captured in a mental life narrative you have been writing since adolescence, remembering and exploring key chapters and events in your life is an important part of developing a sense of authenticity.

Like the author of a novel, you can edit and rewrite chapters in your life narrative to create more positive understandings of troubling events or difficult experiences, which will strengthen your sense of self-integrity.

FURTHER READING

Exceptional: Build Your Personal Highlight Reel and Unlock Your Potential by Daniel M. Cable: This book is packed with research-based insights about how to craft a more authentic and positive sense of self-worth.

Transcend: The New Science of Self-Actualization by Scott Barry Kaufman: The author integrates contemporary science and Maslow's famous hierarchy of needs into an exploration of how to become more authentic.

Wiser Than Me with Julia Louis-Dreyfus: This podcast offers a series of fascinating and insightful life narratives from a variety of compelling women.

Master of Change: How to Excel When Everything Is Changing—Including You by Brad Stulberg: Pundits say change is the only constant, and this book offers practical advice on how to remain authentic as you navigate changes in your personal life and the world around you.

CHAPTER EIGHT

Dedicated Practices

Living Out Core Values

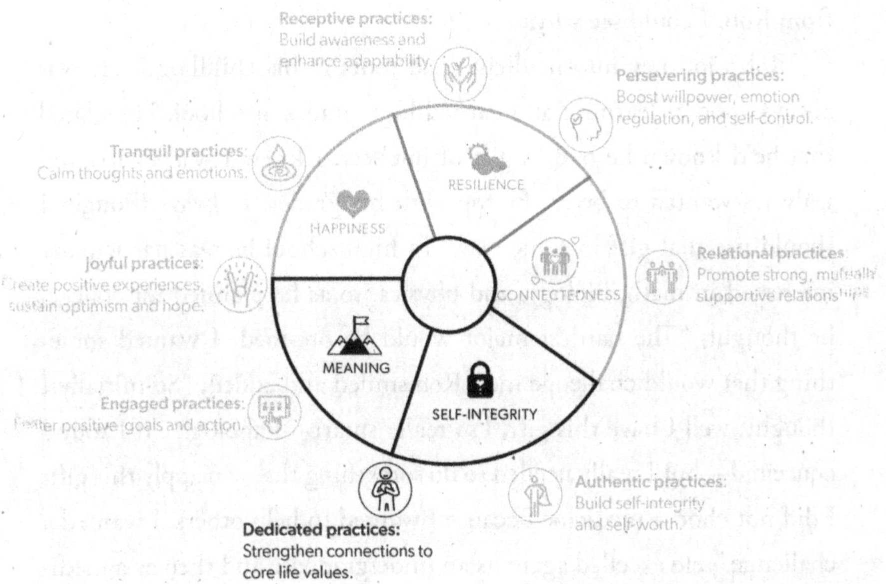

When I walked into Rob's office, he looked more like an off-duty forest ranger than the chief radiologist of one of the Midwest's largest hospitals. Dressed in a faded flannel shirt, well-worn chinos, and rugged boots, he seemed better suited for a cabin in the woods instead of a room filled with medical books. Rob welcomed me warmly with a soft smile and gentle handshake, and encouraged me to sit on a comfortable couch. His demeanor was affable and kind. Our meeting was part of a large research project I was conducting on how people find deeply meaningful work, and Rob had generously scheduled ninety minutes for our interview. Throughout our conversation he listened attentively and made me feel I had his full attention. His responses to my questions were thoughtful and engaging. The hospital's chief medical officer had told me his patients raved about the care they received from Rob. I could see why.

Rob's journey into medicine had roots in his childhood. He was always good at learning and earned high grades at school. He related that he'd known he had "a gift of intellect. I knew I was smart, and I always wanted to be at the top with my grades. I always thought I should use that gift in some way." In high school he was particularly interested in math, biology, and physics, so as he planned for college, he thought, "The hardest major would be pre-med. I wanted something that would challenge me." Rob smiled and added, "So initially I thought, well I have this gift, I'm really smart—I apologize if I sound conceited—but I really needed to do something that can apply this gift. I did not choose medicine because I wanted to help others. I wanted a challenge." He excelled again as an undergraduate and then as a medical school student, always striving to be "at the top." And he was. When it was time to apply for residencies, Rob decided that internal medicine was his first choice. Like most med students, he applied for residencies in several specialties, but felt confident his record of success would lead him where he wanted to go.

But Rob experienced a significant setback: He didn't get his first choice of residency. Harder still, he had to take a residency in radiology, which was "one of my last choices," doing mammography, "the one part of radiology I really wanted to avoid. I didn't have a passion for it." During that time another unexpected experience occurred: His mother developed breast cancer. Her physician was "just a technician, none of the caring side. He just did the procedures and never really talked with my mom about what was happening, what her choices were." As a result, "she declined traditional medical treatment . . . which I found exasperating and it just really threw me." When Rob began his residency in radiology, his mother's cancer became worse. He tried desperately to convince her to change doctors, "to take control of her situation and make better decisions." She did not. Within a few months the cancer took her life.

That was a turning point for him. "That residency that I didn't want turned out to be amazingly lucky . . . It changed everything. Doing mammography, I finally saw that it was the caring part of medicine that I was really drawn to." He paused for a moment, then said, "My mom's struggles made me realize what was important. I knew then that the helping-others side of medicine was the most important thing to me." Rob remembered, "I was a little surprised because previously I thought it was the intellectual, technical side of medicine where I would excel." So, he decided to become a radiologist and focus his practice on mammography even though "it's the most litigious area of medicine. But instead of sitting in a room, I'd be out talking with the patients, helping them make better decisions about their health, helping them understand what is happening to them."

Rob continued to excel in his work, which earned him several promotions and ultimately led to his appointment as chief radiologist, the pinnacle of a medical career. That achievement was not something he had sought, even though "before my residency and my mother's struggles it was the thing I wanted most." But by discovering that one of his core values was helping others, Rob made a significant shift in his career that, as he said, "made all the difference in how things unfolded." He ended our conversation by saying:

> Ultimately as I sit here now, I have come almost full circle and I feel that the helping-others side of it is everything to me now. I have been blessed to be in a situation where I realize that I can truly make a difference and I love that part of it. I begin every day at work reminding myself of that. And, after a particularly bad day, I take time to be grateful that I can really help people. My life is more meaningful than I ever thought it could be.

While Rob had to go through hardships and setbacks to discover his core values and find a path to meaning in life, you can use wise, dedicated practices to strengthen yours. Dedicated practices can help you clarify and embrace your core values and beliefs. They can build your capacity to live out your values, day by day, in all of the important areas of your life; strengthen your connection to something of deep significance; and help you connect with other people in ways that sustain your sense of meaning.

In this chapter I share the insights science offers about how to find and live a more meaningful life, along with some of the wise practices that can strengthen your capacity to do so. Religious and spiritual traditions are also authoritative sources of insight and instruction, and, as I will describe, research shows that these can be immensely helpful. If you have a strong affiliation to such a tradition, I encourage you to rely on its teachings and practices.

Building Blocks of Meaning in Life

In chapter two I presented the consensus view among scholars that experiencing meaning in life arises from three constituents: a belief that there is inherent value in life and that your own life has value and importance (significance); a sense that you are able to contribute to important life aspirations (purpose); and an understanding of what life is truly about that makes existence comprehensible, especially in the face of the uncertainties and difficulties of life (certitude). A fourth element for many people is experiencing a connection with something sacred that is "greater than and more important than" themselves, something they often understand to be divine or in some way transcendent to or "beyond" our normal, everyday material world (spirituality).

Researchers have identified four building blocks for creating a strong sense of meaning in life: clarifying and claiming core values, living out core values through aspirational goals, experiencing meaning through connections with others, and having self-transcendent experiences.

There are certainly other ways of finding and living meaningfully—again, religious and spiritual traditions can be an important source of wisdom—but our focus here is on what science offers.

Core Values

Core values are the guiding principles in our lives.[1] They define the things we care about the most. Legendary psychologist Gordon Allport described them as "ultimate concerns," because they establish the "principles that the individual regards as of ultimate importance in [their] own life, and as having to do with what [the person] regards as permanent or central in the nature of things."[2]

Core values underlie our conceptions of what is true, excellent, and noble, and so they orient us toward what it means to live a good, virtuous, worthwhile life. These conceptions form the interpretive framework we need for purpose, significance, and certitude. Purpose is core values in action. It is a sense that our life has direction that is guided and inspired by personal values and beliefs. These conceptions of a good life also give rise to our sense of significance, our understanding of what makes life itself precious—and our life, in particular, valuable. The frameworks animated by core values help us grapple with life's big questions and make sense of the unfolding experiences of our life and the lives of people we care about, which ground us in a sense of certitude.

I have emphasized that we have to figure out and claim our core values for ourselves, but in doing so we often need to draw upon outside sources of wisdom. One such source of insight is learning from the lives of people we admire, and this simple practice, which I have used in a variety of settings, has proven to be very helpful to people as they clarify their own values.

REFLECT ON PEOPLE YOU ADMIRE

When we admire someone, we see them as an exemplar of what it means to live a good, worthy life. We see in them and their actions reflections of the things that matter most to them. And what creates our feelings of admiration is a sense of resonance and deep agreement with those most important things. In other words, whether we realize it or not, the things that matter most to those we admire are also some of the things that matter most to us.

Begin this practice by selecting at least five people you admire. These should be people you know well, and they do not need to be famous or well known. For instance, my paternal grandfather, Glenn Bloom, is one of the people I admire most. For each person, write what you admire about them. Be as specific as you can. You should choose people about whom you know important details. Be sure to include people you know personally: a friend, relative, teacher, or coach. The people you know really well are the best choices. You can use a famous person whom you don't know personally, but you need to know enough about them so you can describe what you admire about that person.

Try to write at least one full page of description of why you find this person admirable. This is another reflective discovery practice, so at this point you just need some initial, top-of-your-head thoughts and insights. Follow this process for all five or more people you have chosen.

Then, look for patterns across your descriptions. What are the common things you admire? Look especially for the core values that are reflected in those admirable things. What values do you see revealed in these people's lives? You will almost certainly have insights into the things they did that reveal how they lived out those values, so take note of those as well. Both of these discoveries—into the values themselves and the way people enacted those values—will provide important insights for you about your own core values.

The next part of this practice is to begin describing your values. The Values in Action Institute (www.viacharacter.org) offers a list that might help you get started. Your goal here is to identify five to seven values that you feel are most important to you. You will likely feel an affinity toward more than these, but work to winnow your list down to the five to seven most important.

Last, describe each value in detail. What does it mean to you? Why is it important to you? How might you enact or live out that value in your life? What would be different in the lives of people you know or in the world around you if you lived out that value? The goal here is to define each in enough detail that you can say to yourself, "*This* is one of my core values and I understand what it means to me."

Author and life coach Brad Stulberg endorses the importance of core values throughout life, but especially during periods of life change. "Core values," he writes, "play an important role during periods of change, disorder, and uncertainty. When you feel the ground shifting underneath you, when you don't know your next move, you can ask yourself, how might I move in the direction of my core values?"[3] His advice reflects a second principle from research about strengthening your sense of meaning in life: Pursue aspirational life goals.

Aspirational Life Goals

A second building block for fostering a strong sense of meaning in life is enacting your core values by pursuing major life goals that are self-concordant. That somewhat clunky research term refers to goals that enact your core values. Psychiatrist and Holocaust survivor Viktor Frankl affirmed this as well, claiming, "What man actually needs is not a tensionless state . . . but rather a striving and struggling for a worthwhile goal, a freely chosen task."[4]

We will explore goals more deeply in chapter nine, but here I want to share research on the motivations behind goals.[5] There are two basic kinds of goals: those that are intrinsically motivated (we pursue them because we value the objective or goal) and those that are extrinsically motivated (we pursue them to gain external rewards like social status, material possessions, and awards, or because of social pressures imposed on us like following rules, meeting someone else's demands, or fitting in to social groups). When we pursue intrinsically motivating goals, we feel we have freely chosen to do so. We are guided and motivated by our commitment to the goals. They make us feel alive, energized, and authentic in our actions because they are expressions of what matters most to us.

By contrast, when we pursue extrinsically motivated goals, we feel pushed, coerced, or in some other way externally pressured to pursue them. We pursue social status, for example, because we want to feel "better" or more special than other people in some way. We conform to social pressures because we feel compelled to measure up to social standards. We pursue money because we see it as a marker of success. Even when we value the outcomes of extrinsic goals, the feelings of satisfaction we experience from achieving them tend to be ephemeral, so we often find ourselves craving more: more money, more status, more success. Studies show that emphasizing materialistic goals over intrinsic ones tends to undermine wellbeing.[6] A meta-analysis (a powerful statistical methodology that combines data from many studies to gain more precise results) of 105 studies involving more than 70,000 people found that pursuing self-concordant goals was positively linked with happiness, satisfaction with life, and a positive sense of meaning.[7] Pursuing goals related to obtaining objectives like money, status, fame, and beauty was linked to unhappiness and greater incidences of depression and anxiety. This study also found that choosing to prioritize extrinsically motivating goals over self-concordant goals was linked to lower life satisfaction and weaker experiences of meaning and purpose.

We all have to pursue some extrinsic goals in life like earning sufficient income, following important rules, and owning up to our responsibilities, and sometimes these achievements and successes are good for us. We feel great when we earn good grades, receive an award, or get a raise in salary at work. And sometimes extrinsic goals are important parts of striving toward self-concordant goals. For example, I was told I had to earn a PhD at a top-ranked university to become a professor, and I had to achieve tenure so I could engage in my long-term study of wellbeing. The main point is to understand what is motivating your major life goals, the ones that form the direction and purpose of your life. Studies consistently find that pursuing intrinsically motivated, self-concordant goals (as opposed to extrinsically motivated goals) is beneficial for our wellbeing in many ways: We are happier, more satisfied with our jobs and our lives, more eager to engage in personal growth, and more capable of learning new things; have greater self-worth; and experience our lives as more meaningful and fulfilling.[8]

Research by University of Missouri psychologist Ken Sheldon, one of the leading experts on self-concordant goals, suggests that what is important for our wellbeing is finding a balance between self-concordant and extrinsic goals. He frames this around the idea of life balance. Customarily, when people think about life balance, they imagine an ideal allocation of time spent at work and on things outside of work. Sheldon proposes that the problem may not be too much time at work, but too little time spent on self-concordant goals. His Life Balance Inventory can be a wise way to find the balance you need.

A LIFE BALANCE INVENTORY

This is another practice that builds on the Map Your Days exercise. It is best done on paper. I recommend a large, poster-sized piece of paper so you have plenty of room. Make four columns and title them as follows:

1. Areas where I spend my time
2. Amount of time I actually spend on an area
3. Amount of time I want to spend on the area
4. Importance of this area

For the first column, think of a normal, seven-day week and list the major activity areas where you spend time: work, family, sleep, household activities, recreation, community, personal relationships, and so forth.

Move to the second column and fill in the amount of time you actually spend in each area. Think of more than just time; also consider where you give your energy and effort. A supportive person can help you be accurate with your activity areas and time allocations. You now have a map of where you spend your time.

Take a break for a day or two to let your mind clear. Then return to your grid and map out what an ideal or at least better week would look like for you. In the third column, answer these questions: Where do you want to spend your time? What areas of life are the most important and should receive your best efforts? What is a more ideal amount of time to spend in each area? You will most likely see some differences in the actual versus ideal amounts. Where those differences exist, take time to reflect on the reasons underlying those imbalances. Again, conversations with your support person can be helpful for digging into the reasons.

The last step, in the fourth column, is to write next to each point in the third column an "I" if your engagement in that area is mostly for intrinsic reasons or an "E" if it is mostly for extrinsic reasons. Then, look for insights into how you might tip the balance more favorably toward "I" entries.

Of course, the real last step is to use these responses to change how you spend your time. Remember to do this one step at a time. Make one change, and live with it for a while to see how it goes. Then make another. Bit by bit, you can make wholesale changes to orient your days around mostly self-concordant goals and activities.

Meaningful Connections

I am often asked if religious people have higher wellbeing. The answer is, "It depends." Religious people don't have higher wellbeing when they believe in a wrathful, judgmental God, when their beliefs are so restrictive or unrealistic that they can never measure up to them, or when their religious beliefs cause them to be highly judgmental of other people. When we judge others harshly, we activate negative internal judgments, which can cause us to think poorly about ourselves.

Religious people do have higher wellbeing when they believe in a kind and loving God, when their beliefs encourage them to be accepting of their human frailties and others', and when their religious orientation helps them live a good and worthwhile life.[9] The two primary ways that religiosity seems to lead to higher wellbeing is by (1) providing a system of teachings, beliefs, and doctrines that help people clarify and live out core values and (2) creating communities in which people with the same values can form and maintain strong relationships and provide support for each other in myriad ways. Religious and spiritual beliefs can also create a sense of significance by providing ways for people to envision how they are connected to an infinite being, essence, or power that also gives shape to their sense of meaning and purpose.[10]

For both the religious and nonreligious, experiences of meaning in life are often found and created through relationships with others. Parenthood, caring for a loved one who is ill or injured, and experiencing love from a valued other can help us gain clarity about what matters most in life. In addition, for many people the perception that their life matters depends heavily on the belief that their actions have helped make the world a better place for others. Our close relationships also help us restore meaning during tumultuous times. When life challenges us, we often turn to close others to make sense of the situation.

Another relational pathway to meaning is through the experience of a shared reality.[11] This is the perception that you and close others have similar core values. These experiences happen when you feel you share common attitudes, feelings, and opinions about important things in life. You "see the world in the same way." The listening principles and practices we explored in chapter six are wise ways to develop shared reality.

Still another wise practice for fostering shared reality is experiences of nostalgia.[12]

NOSTALGIA

Nostalgia is a sentimental remembering of meaningful past experiences. During these reminiscences, you reexperience aspects of a significant event and activate positive emotions like warmth, love, optimism, hope, and connectedness with important others. As we will learn in chapter ten on joyful practices, positive emotions like these are, in and of themselves, uplifting.[13] They boost happiness and resilience. They also create the *feeling* that life is good and meaningful.[14] Because nostalgia anchors these feelings in a specific memory, we have "inside knowledge" that makes these feelings of meaningfulness seem real to us. We experience them as evidence that there are real reasons our life has meaning. And they are also a subtle but powerful form of encouragement: "I've had meaningful experiences in the past so I will have them again."

We treasure nostalgic memories and seek out cues to them in the songs we listen to, the movies and TV shows we watch, the books we read, and even the things we buy. (Consider the popularity of "retro" products.) Nostalgia can also be prompted by smells, pictures, and other in-the-moment experiences that remind us of the past.

To practice nostalgia, bring to mind a fond memory from your past. As we have done in other practices, try to create a rich description of where this event happened, the important people that were present, and how the event unfolded. Also recall how that experience affected you and how It made you feel. Then take a moment to reflect on what made that event important. You may not be able to describe this in detail, but at least bring to mind some of the broad themes or reasons that make this such a special memory. Look for the core values that were expressed in this experience. The lists of values presented earlier in this chapter can help if you need some ideas. Consider ending with a physical expression that honors the meaningfulness of this experience, like placing your hand over your heart or giving thanks for it.

Shared nostalgic experiences are particularly beneficial: We feel our experiences are affirmed and validated by important others, which boosts their positive effects. You can follow a similar process with another person, ideally someone who was part of the nostalgic memory. These shared moments, even very brief ones, are beneficial in our everyday lives, but they are especially important when we are facing life challenges and difficulties. We feel lifted up and anchored, once again, in some of the most important things in our lives.

Nostalgic reminiscing is something most of us naturally do from time to time, and now you know how to use those experiences to enhance your wellbeing. You can also help others do the same. At its core, this wise practice involves being more intentional about focusing on what makes fond memories meaningful. This is how you can experience the wellbeing benefits those memories contain.

Prosocial behaviors—acts that promote or protect others' wellbeing—are also a relational pathway to meaning.[15] Much of the meaning Rob experiences in his work comes from the many ways he can care for his patients. Health researchers have consistently found positive links between such behaviors and the longevity of both help givers and receivers, partly through the way they increase experiences of meaning in both parties.[16] A meta-analysis of 126 studies including nearly 200,000 people found that acts of kindness boosted authenticity, a sense of meaning and purpose in life, and the self-worth of both the kindness givers and receivers.[17]

For years I have seen bumper stickers that encourage us to "practice random acts of kindness." While I appreciate the underlying sentiment, something is missing or confused in that advice. We should be intentional about practicing acts of kindness, with both people we know and those we don't know. Perhaps that is what "random" is meant to convey—be kind to everyone. Acts of kindness, both small and big, are readily available ways to engage in prosocial behaviors and build a sense of positive connections with others, well known to us and not. We experience a greater sense of meaning in life through the positive connections we have, from transient encounters to lifelong loving relationships.

INTENTIONAL ACTS OF KINDNESS

Acts of kindness are prosocial behaviors that strengthen our sense that life is significant. Both small acts of kindness (a genuinely warm greeting, a sincere offer of gratitude, holding the door for someone as you enter a public building) and larger acts (volunteering, caring for someone who is ill, helping a friend move homes) make us and the people we are kind to happier, more resilient, and more connected.

You can engage in intentional acts of kindness in many different ways. Offer an expression of gratitude to the waitstaff at a restaurant or a store clerk. When he travels by airplane, a friend of mine always thanks the TSA agents for "keeping us safe." Other examples include allowing a driver merging in traffic to get in front of you and saying hello as you pass someone in a hallway.

Of course, there are bigger acts of kindness you can offer: sending a card of encouragement to someone facing a difficult situation, giving a thoughtful gift, making a meal for family or friends, helping a coworker, or sitting with a grieving friend.

The key is to adopt an attitude of kindness. Be intentional about looking for opportunities to be kind.

The practices in chapter six are also wise ways of strengthening your experience of meaning through the important relationships in your life. You might bundle capitalizing and nostalgia as you reminisce about a great memory, or practice gratitude along with forgiveness as you revisit a difficult time with someone you love.

Self-Transcendent Experiences

Columbia University psychologist Lisa Miller, who has conducted pioneering research into the science of spirituality, writes:

> Each of us is endowed with a natural capacity to perceive a greater reality and consciously connect to the life force that moves in, through, and around us. Whether or not we participate in a spiritual practice or adhere to a faith tradition, whether or not we identify as religious or spiritual, our brain has a natural inclination toward and docking station for spiritual awareness. The awakened brain is the neural circuitry that allows us to see the world more fully and thus enhance our individual, societal, and global wellbeing.[18]

This capacity for spiritual awareness in turn creates the capacity for us to have self-transcendent experiences (STEs), moments in which our sense of self takes a back seat and other aspects are enhanced: our attention to and appreciation of the value of other people, the meaningfulness of life, or the things that matter most to us.[19] A hallmark of STEs like inspiration, wonder, and awe is feeling a deep connectedness to something of immense significance—God, the Universe, Infinite Love, the Divine. While these experiences are profoundly moving in themselves, they also lead to significant increases in the meaningfulness of one's life.[20]

In his groundbreaking studies of awe, University of California, Berkeley, psychologist Dacher Keltner defines it as "the feeling of being in the presence of something vast that transcends your current understanding of the world . . . In evoking awe, it reveals that our current knowledge is not up to the task of making sense of what we have encountered. And so, in awe, we go in search of new forms of understanding. Awe is about our relation to the vast mysteries of life."[21] Experiencing awe helps us move beyond the intense busyness of our daily life and free ourselves from mundane trivialities. People report that these experiences open them to seeing, sensing, and understanding deep truths about the meaning of life. Awe also promotes a strong and positive sense of connectedness with other people.[22] And experiences of awe have significant health and wellbeing benefits, including reducing stress levels, boosting happiness, and fostering a sense of peacefulness.[23]

Collective effervescence, a deep sense of unity and joy with a group of people, is one way to evoke awe. It can happen during religious or spiritual gatherings, at a sporting event or live musical performance, or when you hike to an amazing vista with family and friends. Experiences in nature, like witnessing a beautiful sunset, literally stopping to smell the roses, or being in a forest, are also common awe-inspiring experiences. Studies show that even incidental contact with nature can be beneficial. An eighteen-year study of over one hundred thousand city dwellers in the United Kingdom found that people living closer to green spaces reported less mental distress.[24] When people moved closer to natural settings, experiences of mental distress declined, but when they moved farther away, these experiences became more common.[25]

Another STE is moral elevation, which arises from being inspired by another person's courage, kindness, or strength.[26] Stories of moral exemplars, heroes, and people who have risked their safety to help another person touch us deeply because they evoke awe and admiration. Studies show that moral elevation strengthens our understanding of our core values and inspires us to live them out.[27]

We can be inspired by watching movies, reading books, listening to podcasts, or otherwise witnessing a person who has led or is leading a morally exemplary life. Examples for me include movies like *Dead Poets Society*, *Good Will Hunting*, and *Invictus*; Tracy Kidder's biographies of Paul Farmer and Jim O'Connell; and some of the interviews Julia Louis-Dreyfus conducts with noted women in their seventies and up on her podcast, *Wiser Than Me*.

This next practice is one of my favorites because it takes me out of my usual analytic thinking style and opens me to new insights while strengthening the joy I experience in living out my core values.

MORAL EXEMPLARS

This practice is similar to the reflect on people you admire practice in that it creates a pathway for you to explore more deeply your core values and what makes your life meaningful. Select a movie, book, or other piece of media about someone you regard as a moral exemplar. Here's the key: As you read or watch, allow yourself to *feel* the inspiration, to be moved and uplifted by what you experience. Pause occasionally to reflect on what you are experiencing. You might add in the wise practice of emotional granularity by crafting a rich description of the thoughts and feelings you experienced. This is a way to develop deeper insights into meaning and then move to thinking about your core values.

When you finish your chosen media, reflect again on the entire experience and be especially open to thoughts and insights about what makes that person awesome to you. Reflect on the core values you share and remind yourself of the ways you see them living them out. This pairing of moral elevation with contemplation about your values strengthens your understanding of and commitment to those values. You can enhance the wellbeing benefits by sharing your thoughts and feelings with a close other, or by writing down some thoughts about your experience. Again here, the core of this wise practice is being more intentional about looking for and reflecting on the meaning you can find in the lives and actions of your moral exemplars.

STEs help us imagine a new and better future, one in which we grow more fully into our best selves, experience stronger connections with others, and see ways we can contribute to making the world a better place. They intrinsically motivate us to live a life of value and purpose. And they help us *feel*, in deep and profound ways, the meaningfulness of our life.

KEY INSIGHTS

Meaning in life arises from a sense that your life is significant, that it has an important purpose or purposes, and that there is an underlying existential order to existence.

Clarifying and committing to your core values is foundational for strengthening and sustaining a sense of meaning in life.

A sense of purpose in life arises from building your major life priorities and commitments around your core values, and from integrating them into your daily activities.

Our connections and relationships with significant others are important pathways for expressing and experiencing meaning.

STEs of awe and wonder can strengthen and deepen your experience of meaning.

FURTHER READING

Awe: The New Science of Everyday Wonder and How It Can Transform Your Life by Dacher Keltner: A heartfelt and wise book written by a leading expert on STEs and wellbeing.

The Awakened Brain: The New Science of Spirituality and Our Quest for an Inspired Life by Lisa Miller: An inspiring exploration of religiosity and spirituality.

Freely Determined: What the New Psychology of the Self Teaches Us About How to Live by Kennon M. Sheldon: The psychology of self-concordance written by a highly accomplished researcher.

Your favorite spiritual resource. Among mine are collections of poetry and books about religious mystics.

CHAPTER NINE

Engaged Practices

Pursuing Life-Enriching Goals

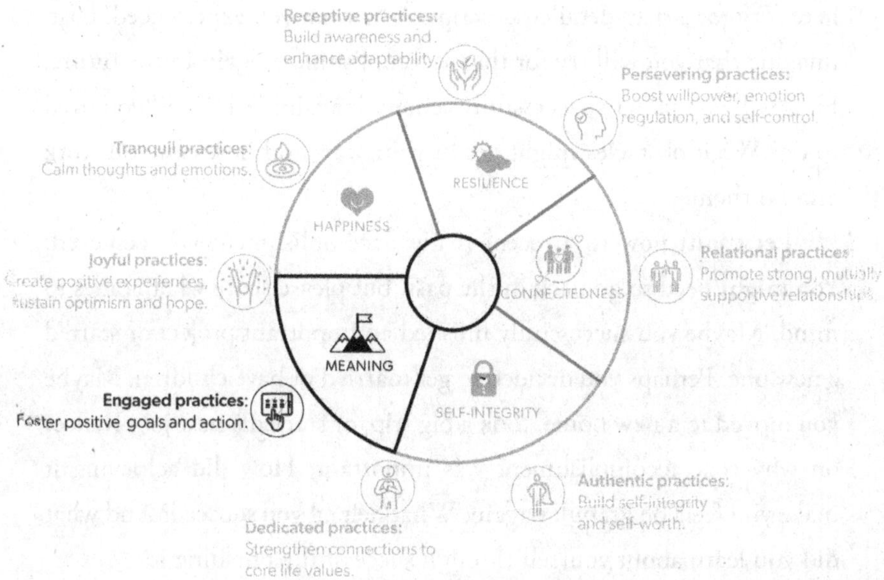

This chapter begins with a story about an individual, as other chapters have, but this time the individual is you! I invite you to engage in a mental role-playing activity with me. Tell me about one thing you accomplished today that you are happy about. It can be anything. Maybe you wanted to get up early and you did. Or maybe you needed to buy groceries and successfully did so. Or perhaps you wanted to have dinner with family or friends and you enjoyed that time together. Maybe you went to the gym or got the oil changed in your car. Or perhaps you wanted to read a book and are accomplishing that right now.

With that accomplishment in mind, please take a moment to share why you chose to go after it. Why was it important to you? Try to be as specific as you can about the underlying reasons or motivations. Now share what it felt like to finish it. Practice emotional granularity here: Try for a rich, detailed description of what you experienced. Last, imagine that you will try for that accomplishment again in the future. How will you plan to successfully achieve it again? What will you need to do? What obstacles might get in your way, and how can you work around them?

Let's shift now to a recent major accomplishment you achieved. You might need to go back in the past, but please share what comes to mind. Maybe you successfully finished an important project or started a new one. Perhaps you decided to get married or have children. Maybe you moved to a new home, took a big trip, or started a new job. Reflect on why that accomplishment was important. How did achieving it make you feel? Be granular again. What helped you succeed? And what did you learn about yourself through successfully pursuing it?

Each one of these accomplishments was a goal and, like most good goals, they shared some common characteristics:

- They were specific; you knew what you wanted to accomplish.
- They were realistic; you had the capacity to achieve the goal.
- They could be planned; you were able to map out a way to achieve them, or at least take the first steps toward attaining them.
- They were adaptable; you could change how you were pursuing them as circumstances dictated.
- And, most importantly, they were meaningful; it was important to you to achieve each of these accomplishments.

Goals are mental representations of future outcomes or objectives you want to attain and that you strive, with some degree of persistence, to reach. We pursue all kinds of goals, from big ones like searching for a new job, committing to a life partner, or deciding to become a parent, to smaller, everyday goals like deciding to start a new exercise regimen, planning to buy groceries for the week, or getting together with friends for a dinner.

Why do goals matter for wellbeing? Award-winning author Annie Dillard offers one of the most succinct and poignant answers: "How we spend our days is, of course, how we spend our lives."[1] This important philosophical point has immense practical relevance. Our lives unfold one day at a time, and our days are structured mostly around the goals toward which we dedicate time, attention, and effort. So, the goals we are spending time on create the lives we experience ourselves as living. Our lives seem meaningful when most of our daily pursuits are important to us. Remember that the most important part of happiness is life satisfaction, which is your evaluation of how your life is unfolding. To feel good about how your life is going, it's important to spend your days on the right kind of goals, those that are expressions of your core values. What matters most are the big goals, the ones that give shape and substance to your life.

Engaged and dedicated practices are very tightly linked. Dedicated practices help you clarify and live out your core values. Engaged practices help you pursue the goals you really want to go after, rather than those that other people impose or that in some other way creep into your days. When it comes to boosting and sustaining meaning, pursuing goals that are expressions of your core values is key.

If this is the area of wellbeing where your needs are greatest, begin by stepping back. Take a look at how you are spending your days. What goals are you dedicating most of your time to? Which goals are life enriching? Which ones are most life depleting? If your life has become too stressful, or if you feel your life is headed in the wrong direction, you likely need to start by figuring out which goals you need to stop pursuing. This might not be an easy step, but it is likely to be an essential one. The only way to shed the stress and get your life back on track is to stop doing the things that are making your life intolerable. Then, you have room to build more life-enriching goals into your days. You might use the "Life Balance Inventory" practice from chapter eight. Or you might audit your to-do lists or schedule to see how you are spending your days.

AUDITING YOUR TO-DO LISTS AND SCHEDULE

↶ This practice is another variation of Map Your Days. Your to-do lists and schedule are ways you clarify and perhaps organize the goals you are going after. When I ask people about how things are going, most people tell me they are too busy. And when

I ask what that means, they say they have too many things to do, emphasis on *have*. When I then ask them what they would rather be doing, most people can come up with a list. The perhaps not-so-obvious conclusion is they are not spending their days going after the goals they really value.

Begin by taking a look at your to-dos or schedule and making a list of the major goals represented there. An item on your to-do list or an event on your schedule is a reflection of some underlying goal. You might have to dig a little to surface the goal, and it might take some candid reflection to be willing to admit you have one or more of those goals, but they are there. Make a second column on your list of goals and quickly assess whether each is an intrinsic goal or an extrinsic one. Notice the kinds of goals on your list. How do you feel about those goals? How many are extrinsic? Make a third column and describe the reward, pressure, rule, or external force for each extrinsic goal. In that third column, write the core value that is motivating each intrinsic goal.

Take time to reflect on what you are learning about how you are spending your days. Where is change needed? What goals should you stop striving for? Which ones should you eliminate, and for which will this be difficult? What makes stopping those goals difficult? Where could you swap out a less important goal for one you really want to work toward? This is another practice where the input and insights of a close other can be very helpful.

Modern life can make it very difficult to fill your days with life-enriching goals. Georgetown professor Cal Newport has written extensively and expertly about what he calls "the dehumanizing grip of pseudo-productivity," which for many working professionals has created a "relentless overload that's wearing us down." He digs into the underlying motivation, "a belief that 'good' work requires increasing busyness—faster responses to email and chats, more meetings, more tasks, more hours. But when we look closer at this premise, we fail to find a firm foundation."[2] In other words, the way many of us are spending our work days is creating untenable and unfulfilling lives.

Reading Newport's thought-provoking book, I remembered the movie *Jerry Maguire*. It struck me how well a film made almost thirty years ago captures the experiences of so many people today. It opens with Maguire writing a mission statement in a hotel room. He experiences an epiphany: He is deeply dissatisfied with his work and imagines a more meaningful alternative. He writes about his vision for a new way of working and concludes:

> A life is not worth living if you are sleepwalking through it. Because that is what feels like death . . . It is the feeling of sleepwalking. Of others living life around you, keeping their fists tightly wound around whatever dollars they can muster, caring little more than nothing about those around you . . . We can take control of our lives, we can quit sleepwalking, we can say—right now, these are our lives, it is time to start living it.[3]

That statement becomes the catalyst for profound changes in Maguire's life. He finds stronger connections with important people and more meaningful work because he started spending his days on life-enriching goals, striving to achieve things that really mattered to him. This movie captures both the difficulties and the importance of knowing what matters most and building your life pursuits on those things.

In this chapter we will explore insights about how you can also make better choices about the goals you pursue. I will share wise practices you can use to make both small and big changes to how you spend your days. How you spend your days is, of course, how you are spending your life.

The Elements of Life-Enriching Goals

Achievable goals are specific, realistic, plannable, and adaptable. If we want to make goal attainment more likely, we need to structure our pursuits around these four elements. Life-enriching goals add one more element: They are meaningful. They follow the principles from chapter eight. When people report that their life has purpose, it's because they spend most of their days striving toward life-enriching goals.

This section might seem a bit like a tutorial about how to set and achieve goals, but intentionality is essential here. To make life meaningful, you need to be intentional about choosing the goals you want to go after. You also have to be intentional about setting goals you can achieve. To do so, you need to know and apply the elements of achievable goals. Let's work through these elements.

Specific means the outcome you seek is described in enough detail that it creates a clear objective or target. For example, "lose weight" isn't specific enough. "Lose five pounds" is better and "lose five pounds in six weeks" is better still. "Get a college degree" is too broad, "get a bachelor's degree in psychology" is better, and "get a bachelor's degree in psychology from a state university in four years" is even better. The point here is to be clear enough about what outcome you want to achieve so that you can create a plan for how to go after it. If your goal is "get a better job," you need to be more specific about what "better" means for you. You might define a better job as one that is in your current field and industry, but that also allows you more free time. You might add other criteria, like the new job should pay as well as your current one and allow you to live in your current home.

Even small goals need to be specific. For a long time, when I needed to get my truck serviced, I would just put a sticky note on my desk saying, "Get the oil changed." Often weeks would go by and the note would still be "reminding me." I had to be more specific: "Call to schedule an oil change for the truck today." Then I could create a more useful reminder: "Truck service scheduled for Wednesday at 2:00 PM."

Realistic means that achieving the goal is possible, both in terms of the outcome itself and your capacity to achieve it. Consider if you have the time, talent (the knowledge, skills, and abilities needed), and temperament (dedication, willingness to persevere) to achieve a particular goal. "Lose sixty pounds in one week" is not a realistic goal for anyone. "Lose ten pounds in a month" might be realistic for some, but you would have to decide whether you have the time and knowledge required to prepare healthy meals and develop an appropriate exercise plan, and the fortitude to stick with your plans. We tend to over- or underestimate our talent and temperament, so getting input and guidance from significant or similar others will help ensure your goals are realistic.

If your goal is specific and realistic, you can map out the steps you need to take to accomplish the goal—in other words, your goal is *plannable*. Planning makes goal achievement more likely than if you just wing it. It helps you ensure that you have included all of the important steps and defined them specifically enough so that you know how to take each one. It allows you to gather the resources you need, including obtaining the help and support of other people, for each step.

Planning also helps you uncover potential obstacles so you can prepare for them. One of those potential obstacles is figuring out how you will keep yourself motivated to work toward a goal. We tend to overestimate how persistent we will be when goal pursuits get tough or boring. A wise practice for planning uses the amazing capacity we have to engage in mental time travel. We can, for example, revisit past events and experience them almost as if they were happening again, and imagine, in detail, future events that might happen.

Mental contrasting practices are one way we can use our capacity for mental time travel to enhance goal planning. We create a rich mental image of a goal we want to achieve, and then contrast and compare it with our current reality, noting the obstacles and impediments that might stand in the way of achieving that desired future state. The key is to create a detailed image of the goal you want to achieve, including being specific about what will be different and better when you attain it, and what will have changed in your life.

Mentally contrasting a hoped-for future against your present reality can help in several ways. It prompts you to form positive expectations of success, which strengthens your motivation to strive for the goal. It boosts your self-confidence to help you achieve the goal. And it helps empower you to overcome obstacles. When people's expectations of success are high, they are more likely to fully commit to and actively pursue their goals. It is especially helpful when you are going after a really important goal, both before you start and also when you run into difficulties.

I taught this mental contrasting practice many times in my MBA and executive education classes. I usually got eye rolls when I shared it, but later on, the eye rollers often told me it was really helpful. It's also a practice you can use on your morning commute, while you are exercising, or during another routine task.

IMAGINING OBSTACLES TO A HOPED-FOR FUTURE

To begin this practice, you might step easy by trying it with a smaller goal. Say, for example, your goal is to finish an important project over the weekend. You imagine as vividly as you can what achieving the goal would be like and what it would mean to you to attain it. Then you shift to imagining your present reality and the obstacles that stand in the way of attaining the goal. Maybe you want to attend a friend's birthday party Saturday night, or you are an avid football fan and there are several big games over the weekend. With those obstacles in mind, shift to thinking about what you can do to overcome them. Remember that one of the obstacles might be your own dwindling motivation. A good way to end is to add the silver lining practice from page 100 and imagine what it will feel like when you accomplish this goal.

A recent study showed how mental contrasting can help overcome obstacles to goal commitment and striving.[4] A major challenge healthcare providers face is getting people to read and follow information that would be beneficial for their physical health. This is especially true when people are at risk for serious health issues. Adopting new health behaviors is a big, important goal that, unfortunately, many find difficult to achieve. Researchers tested mental contrasting with people at high risk for developing melanoma. After confirming that all the participants hoped to be able to adopt healthier behaviors that would mitigate their risk of cancer, the researchers divided participants into a control group and a group that learned the "hoped-for future" mental contrasting practice. The control group was asked to list three reasons why it would be good for anyone with melanoma risk to learn how to manage it better. The mental contrasting group was asked to first reflect on the benefits of learning about melanoma. Then they reflected on their greatest fear about ignoring their risk and considered what they might lose if they ignored it. All participants were then given the opportunity to learn about how to manage their cancer risk. Those in the mental contrasting group were more than twice as likely to take advantage of that opportunity; most importantly, they were also much more likely to follow the health guidance they learned.

We have covered three elements of achievable goals—they are specific, realistic, and plannable. Let's now look at the fourth thing a goal must be: *adaptable*. This means that both your goal and plan for achieving it are flexible enough to accommodate the vicissitudes of life and goal pursuits. An adaptable goal allows you to change the outcome you are striving for. Using my example of getting a new job, you might need to include more industries if acceptable jobs aren't available in your current one. If you want to get a college degree in psychology, you might need to include other universities if you cannot gain admission to your preferred institution. Mental contrasting can help you identify what aspects of the goal you are willing to change. Adaptable plans can be adjusted or tweaked to accommodate shifts in factors that affect your ability to pursue the goal. For example, you might need to adjust the milestones you have set or update your timeline for accomplishing the goal. More often, adaptations are needed to deal with obstacles that arise. In other words, building in some ways you can adapt your goal pursuits for obstacles you might face is a good way to help you deal with the ones you didn't expect.

An often-overlooked aspect of adaptability is being clear about if and when you might stop pursuing a goal. There's a phenomenon called "escalating commitment to a losing course of action" that highlights the fact that once we commit to a goal, we tend to continue striving for it even when success is unlikely or when pursuing the goal has become overly problematic. Specifying when and why you would stop goal-striving is especially important for bigger, more resource-intensive goals. It can be a good way to motivate yourself to keep going when the going gets tough. If you haven't hit your criteria for stopping, then you know you should keep striving. You may just need to adapt how you are going after the goal. Changing tactics can help you find a path around obstacles and create new energy to keep you going.

The fifth element, *meaningful*, is the most important. Building your days around goals that are expressions of your core values may be the hardest part of creating a more meaningful life. You may have to make tough decisions about how you are spending your days. Cal Newport advocates for adopting an approach to choosing and pursuing life goals he calls slow productivity, which, "more than anything else, is a plea to step back from the frenzied activity of the daily grind. It's not that these efforts are arbitrary: our anxious days include tasks and appointments that really do need to get done. But once you realize . . .

that this exhausted scrambling is often orthogonal to the activities that matter, your perspective changes."[5]

"Orthogonal" here means you are focusing on less important goals to the exclusion of those you really care about. And, as Newport convincingly describes, breaking free from this exhausting scramble often means working around or against the cultures that push us into it. His approach is straightforward and very countercultural, beginning with the most important principle: Do fewer things. When our days are too full, we don't have any space to add in life-enriching pursuits. Newport's important advice is that we need to free up space, and the best way to do that is to do less. Stop doing some of the things that make your days stressful. Set more realistic expectations for what you can reasonably achieve and still maintain your wellbeing. And make space for more important things.

When we are locked in "frenzied activity," we are already doing fewer things—we just don't realize we are doing fewer of the things we really value. Being intentional about choosing the few things we really want to do is a very wise practice, but may require tough choices. When I was locked into an unfulfilling job, I finally had to make a big choice: quit or keep slogging. I quit, then went after a more meaningful goal of getting a PhD. It's hard to convey the positive impact of those choices, but at the time both were really difficult. I often shared this story in the courses I taught to business executives. Each time I did, several executives told me they felt locked in their jobs and wanted a way out. A few made a similarly big change, which a former CEO described as "turning my life around." "I didn't know that giving up that prestigious job, the one I thought I could never leave, was the thing I needed to do to finally find meaningful work," he wrote to me in an email. Tough choices, but they can be life-changing.

Pursuing Life-Enriching Goals

Building your days around life-enriching goals is a process of personal growth and change. Three areas of scientific research provide insights into ways you can support and encourage that process. Research on growth mindsets offers insights into how the way we think about the possibility of personal changes influences our capacity to make them. Studies of rituals show how they can be wise ways to reinforce meaningful pursuits. And insights about the importance of social support for living a meaningful life are also applicable for making meaningful life changes.

Mindsets Matter

A mindset is like a theory we hold about the world and how it works. Any mindset is a collection of assumptions that shape how we perceive, interpret, and respond to a particular aspect of life. We have mindsets about many things, such as work, our relationships with important people, and significant life events like becoming a parent and aging. Important here are the mindsets we hold about goals, especially those related to personal changes.

Stanford psychologist Carol Dweck conducted groundbreaking research into how mindsets shape the way we respond to goals.[6] She began with a simple but powerful idea: We can see the human qualities we need to pursue goals—qualities like intelligence, creativity, kindness, and self-control—as innate, hardwired capacities that are locked in from birth. Dweck calls this a fixed mindset. Or, we can adopt a mindset where we view those same capacities as changeable qualities we can develop and improve. She calls this a growth mindset. In Dweck's early work, she found that high school students who struggled to learn new skills or acquire new knowledge did so because they believed that intelligence is innate and they didn't have enough. When students with a fixed mindset performed poorly, they interpreted it as confirming they lacked intelligence. That reinforcement undermined future academic performance further, and these students tended to give up and stop trying.

By contrast, Dweck found that students who believed, or could be convinced, that intelligence is malleable expected they could improve theirs through hard work. They tended to be more self-confident and more likely to persevere in the face of challenges. The performance of these students also improved over time. This mindset change led to a surprising outcome. For many years, scientists thought that IQ was innate and therefore unchangeable. This means your performance on a test would be the same over time. Dweck's finding that students' performance on IQ tests improved after adopting a growth mindset provides a powerful counterclaim.

Since then, studies show that growth mindsets are beneficial for people of all ages. Holding a growth mindset has significant benefits for our capacity to achieve goals: We work harder, persist longer, adapt better, and achieve more when we do.[7] Recent studies indicate that adopting a growth mindset is important for our wellbeing.[8] With a fixed mindset, people tend to internalize mental health challenges as fixed (e.g., "I *am* a depressed or anxious person"), whereas those with a growth mindset tend to externalize those challenges (e.g., "I am *experiencing* depression and I can get better"). Much like perspective shifting and adopting a challenge orientation, adopting the mindset that you can achieve an important goal enhances your capacity to make those positive changes. This is especially true for bigger goals since pursuing them often does entail personal growth.

ADOPT A GROWTH MINDSET

Begin by educating yourself more on the science of mindsets until you are convinced they matter. When I teach this to people they often think it either sounds too good to be true—"Just shifting my mindset can't really make that big of a difference"—or they doubt their capacity to make this change. Reading Carol Dweck's book, or the one by her colleague David Yeager (both of which are listed in Further Reading at the end of this chapter), will provide the scientific evidence that can convince you of the power of a growth mindset and your capacity to adopt one.

Then, consider ways to integrate that mindset into your daily life. Step easy by learning how to apply a growth mindset to a smaller goal like adopting a more intense exercise routine, overhauling your food choices, or committing to spending more time with your family. Remember that it's called a *growth* mindset: Focus on growing in the areas that matter to you. Success, failure—you will likely experience both. Focus on how you can get better, and try to identify several possible areas of growth. Or, you might focus on how you can stretch yourself, how you can lean into going after your goal in ways that will help you achieve it.

Once you are actively pursuing your goal, step back occasionally to take note of how you are getting better. For example, notice what you have learned about how to be more effective in your goal pursuits, or where you are better at motivating yourself. Getting feedback from others can be especially helpful because they can often see growth you can't. Practice capitalizing, from chapter six, with these people as well. Celebrate the growth you have achieved, no matter how small it might seem. The subtle power of a growth mindset will build over time as you become more adept at shifting your perspective.

Growth mindsets are important for any personal goal, so they can be helpful in many places on your wellbeing journey. They are also wise ways to practice perspective shifting and build psychological flexibility. I have placed them here because building more meaning into your daily life may be one of the most important and yet also challenging parts of your journey. Adopting a growth mindset will strengthen your confidence and your capacity to fill your days with life-enriching goals.

Use Rituals to Reinforce Meaningful Goals

Rituals are a simple and powerful way to convey meaning.[9] Religious rituals are excellent examples: bowing with hands folded in front of your face, washing hands and feet before entering a sacred space, the four movements of the Sign of the Cross, sitting with hands held out and palms up. A simple set of behaviors, performed in the same way each time, carries deep meaning. Rituals sometimes employ everyday objects—bread, water, incense, a candle—that are also symbols of something significant and important.

Rituals convey and reinforce meaning in several ways.[10] They embody meaning through the movements or actions they entail. Meaning becomes more concrete by performing a ritual. Rituals are also salient reminders of significance. The actions they entail are tactile, tangible reminders of a value or belief. Rituals, because of their simplicity, can be used during even the busiest days. And when used in groups, rituals create and reinforce strong connections among members, reminding them of the core values they share. Because rituals evoke positive emotions, they create intrinsic motivation to live in consonance with the values the ritual symbolizes.

RITUALS

As you work to shape your days and the goals that fill them around your core values, consider creating a ritual to reinforce this change. I have a tattoo on my left forearm of five birds and a red thread connecting them. Each bird represents one of my core values, and the thread represents a poem that is important to me, William Stafford's "The Way It Is." In the morning, I touch the birds, one by one, and say out loud the value each one represents. I pause to reflect on why that value is important to me. I end by reading Stafford's poem. This simple ritual reminds me of my values, strengthens my commitment to living them out, and centers me so that I can be more intentional about how I live each day. I know several people who end their day with the Prayer of Examen and find that, among other benefits, it strengthens their commitment to living out their religious beliefs. And the ritual Renee and her team use to start their work day—reading an inspirational poem or Scripture, practicing mindfulness meditation, and hugging each other—inspires them to continue their good work.

Step Together to Make Life More Meaningful

Recall from chapter eight on dedicated practices that one of the ways religiosity increases wellbeing, according to research studies, is by uniting people around a set of shared values. Religious gatherings and activities are opportunities for members to be reminded of these shared values, taught ways they can live them in their daily lives, and encouraged that living this way is important. In the Quaker tradition, the practice of forming a Clearness Committee is a way for a member who wishes to make a significant change in their life to receive the social support they need.[11] The member selects a group of people they trust to provide insight, support, and encouragement as they work toward the personal growth or life change they seek. The committee engages in "deep listening" as the member shares the change they are considering. The committee members then ask open-ended, probing questions to help the member understand more clearly the nature of the potential change. The member is given the opportunity to respond to these questions, and then together with the committee, they consider whether there are additional questions that need to be explored further. If so, additional meetings are convened until the member has clarity about the change they wish to make.

In my interviews with Quaker leaders, several explained that a Clearness Committee can be formed to support a member through change in several important ways. The committee can serve as a sounding board for the member to think through the change, to help them clarify why it matters, and to support them in dealing with obstacles or solving problems. Committee members can provide ongoing encouragement as the member journeys toward the desired change, and the emotional support, care, and, when necessary, tough love to help the member continue forward.

CLEARNESS COMMITTEE

Consider forming your own support group to journey with you into a more meaningful daily life. You can create a committee to serve any purposes you think will be helpful for you. While the traditional Quaker committee acts as a sounding board to help a member discern a path forward, you might want your committee to be more active in offering advice and guidance, or ongoing support and encouragement, or help in solving problems and working around obstacles. You might ask them to offer tough love when your motivation wanes. You decide what would be helpful.

Select people whom you are relationally close to and people whom you can trust, both in terms of their capacity to be good committee members and their ability to maintain confidentiality. The committee does not have to meet together—you can meet with members individually or in sub-groups—but doing so is a best practice because members can create a stronger support group when they are in the same space.

The purpose of the first meeting is for you to share your core values, hopes, and aspirations for shaping your daily life, important goal pursuits around those values, and any concerns you have about potential obstacles you might face, including your capacity to make the necessary changes. This is also the time for you to share how the members can help you in your journey. Be as specific as possible. If you want their advice, be clear about what kind will be helpful. If you want regular check-ins with them, specify how often and what purpose you want those check-ins to serve. Set up a schedule of committee meetings and their structure. Ideally, during those meetings you will share with the committee the progress you feel you have made, the obstacles you faced, and the specific changes you want to make before the next meeting.

Again, you can design a committee to serve any purposes that will be helpful for you to make what is most likely a significant life change.

KEY INSIGHTS

"How we spend our days is, of course, how we spend our lives." If your days feel busy but unfulfilling, or if life seems to be passing you by, consider doing an audit of your daily goals—you might need to incorporate some that are more life enriching.

Life-enriching goals are specific, realistic, plannable, adaptable, and meaningful.

Adopting a growth mindset enhances your capacity to establish and successfully pursue life-enriching goals.

Rituals can serve as both tangible symbols of your core values and daily reminders of the values you wish to shape your days.

Supportive others are often invaluable to encourage and care for you as you build your days around meaningful goals.

FURTHER READING

Better Days: Tame Your Inner Critic by Neal Allen: A very helpful guide to overcoming perfectionism and other forms of excessive self-criticism.

Mindset: The New Psychology of Success by Carol S. Dweck: This legendary researcher shares powerful insights and practical advice from her decades of research. Another book I wish had been available when my boys were young.

How to Change: The Science of Getting from Where You Are to Where You Want to Be by Katy Milkman: Chock-full of wise practices and scientific insights, this book will help you change your days for the better.

Stretch: Unlock the Power of Less—and Achieve More Than You Ever Imagined by Scott Sonenshein: An engaging, research-based guide for how to break free from the relentless chase after more, more, more.

10 to 25: The Science of Motivating Young People by David S. Yeager: Although this book is oriented toward adults, the practical insights and wise practices can easily be adapted for all ages.

CHAPTER TEN

Joyful Practices

Nourishing Happiness and Meaning

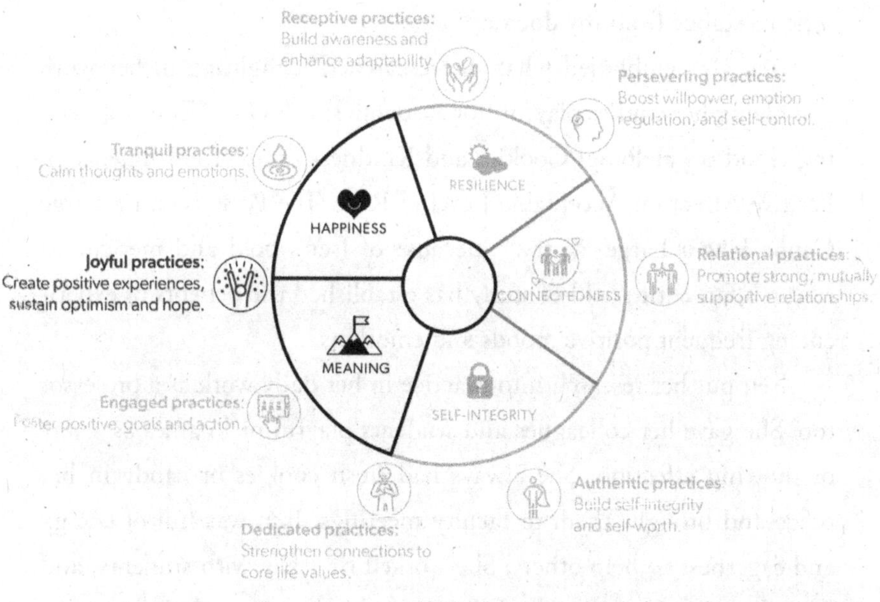

Alice Isen was a pioneering researcher in many respects. She was instrumental in undoing the pernicious dominance of behaviorism in psychology, which equated human behavior with bar-pressing rats. Isen nearly single-handedly established the foundations for what is now known as positive psychology through her groundbreaking research into positive moods and emotions. In 1970 Isen published a landmark study on the "warm glow of success."[1] Using clever techniques and innovative measures, she found that people who were randomly assigned to experience positive feedback were more generous, helpful, and attentive to other people compared to those who were assigned to experience either negative or no feedback. She famously demonstrated that physicians who received an unexpected bag of candy made better medical decisions, something I keep in mind anytime I seek assistance from my doctor.[2]

Isen also embodied what she researched, delighting in her work and giving her studies playful (for academics) titles like "Effect of Feeling Good on Helping: Cookies and Kindness" and "The Influence of Positive Affect on Acceptable Level of Risk: The Person with a Large Canoe Has a Large Worry."[3] Because of Isen's bold and meticulous research, an entire field of study has established the benefits of experiencing frequent positive moods and emotions.

Isen put her research into practice in her daily work as a professor too. She gave her colleagues and students playful nicknames as a way of showing affection. She always had fresh cookies or candy in her office and brought them to faculty meetings. Isen was full of energy and eagerness to help others. She worked tirelessly with students, and earned their admiration and devotion. Her work, and the way she embodied it, created the scientific foundations for joyful practices.

In this chapter we will explore the science of joy, learning about what it is and the pathways through which joyful experiences can nourish wellbeing. I will also share some of the wise practices that have strong research support for being among the best ways to foster joy.

Please keep in mind, however, that many of the wise practices in chapters three through nine have the added benefit of fostering joy. For example, tranquil practices foster the joyful emotions of peacefulness, serenity, and calm. Receptive practices help us learn to see events, other people, and the world around us in more positive ways and increase our capacity to notice and experience everyday joys. Dedicated and engaged practices build a deeper sense of meaning that, in turn, heightens our capacity for joyful experiences like inspiration, wonder, and awe. Let's begin by developing a richer understanding of joy.

Joy Is Fundamental for Wellbeing

Wellbeing researchers agree with philosophers and theologians that joy is a basic constituent of human flourishing. George Vaillant, summarizing key insights from his thirty-five years as director of the Harvard Grant Study (see chapter six), wrote, "We cannot understand human beings unless we understand joy and how joy comes to be."[4] Robert Emmons, a leading wellbeing researcher, writes that joy "is a quality that makes life worth living. Joy is fundamental to human existence and well-being."[5]

While the term "joy" is used by philosophers to denote a virtue and by theologians to describe spiritual enrichment, for social scientists joy is the foundational emotion that is common to experiences like inspiration, hope, awe, exaltation, serenity, optimism, and love. Joy arises when we experience something beautiful, virtuous, profound, or in some other way fundamentally good.

Joy is uplifting; it elevates us and motivates us to respond in a way that enacts or honors it. During experiences of joy, researcher Charles Mathewes writes, "our action, our responsiveness, is solicited, to join in something larger than ourselves, as we are called into true communion with others, in richer, more exuberant life."[6] It reminds us of, connects us to, and calls us to move toward the important things in life. Emmons writes that "joy points beyond itself to something deeply true about human nature and purpose. In true joy, our souls are opened."[7]

Joy is a deeper, richer, and more moving experience than pleasurable emotions like enjoyment, cheerfulness, relaxation, curiosity, and delight. Unlike pleasurable emotions, we can experience joy in the midst of sorrow, pain, and other negative experiences. While grieving a loved one's death, we remember their love and affection, and feel joy. Philosopher and poet Kahlil Gibran famously wrote, "The deeper that sorrow carves into your being, the more joy you can contain."[8]

Joyful emotions strengthen wellbeing in four ways. They are the best pathway to happiness. They build new psychological resources that strengthen our wellbeing. They nourish stronger relationships with others. And they strengthen our sense of self-integrity.

Joy Strengthens Happiness

One of the main stumbling blocks to happiness is that we are not very adept at knowing what makes us happy. Studies show that people tend to mis-predict how good they will feel and how long their happy feelings will last after experiences they think will make them happy, like receiving a windfall of money, scoring well on a test, winning a sports competition, receiving a work promotion, or getting a new car.[9] It's not that we don't feel good after these experiences, it's that those good feelings are often less powerful and more transient than we predicted. The initial thrill of a new car, for example, diminishes after a time, and might even be followed with a taint of buyer's remorse. Right after that big sports win we feel great, but the thrill fades as we focus on an upcoming competition. These kinds of experiences aren't always bad for us; in moderation they can enrich our lives. Pleasure seeking is problematic when it becomes a primary life pursuit.[10] A study of over two hundred thousand people, for example, found that those who pursued pleasurable experiences at high levels also reported lower life satisfaction and felt more boredom in their life.[11]

Researchers have found that the activities that produce the greatest happiness—the greatest positive affect and highest life satisfaction—are those that evoke joy. A seminal study asked 909 women to map their days, charting their major daily activities over the course of two weeks, and then rate how happy they felt doing each one.[12] In order of positivity, the activities that were associated with the greatest happiness and that evoked joyful emotions were intimate relations with their partner, socializing with friends, praying/worshipping/meditating, and caring for their children. The women also reported that participating in the study helped them realize how joy-filled their lives were. Taking time to think about how they spent their time and how they felt about those activities gave them the opportunity to see what really made them happy. Daily life brought them a lot of opportunities to experience joy; they just had to notice and appreciate them.

Therein lies one of the key insights from research. Daily life tends to bring most of us the kinds of joyful experiences that can boost happiness. A connection when you are with someone you love. Being moved by a book, movie, or work of art. Feeling swept away in a spiritual experience. Watching your child's first steps. The serenity in a moment of profound peace. The pride of a job well done. Dinner with people we love, watching a funny movie that brightens our mood, making progress on an important project. We just need to notice and appreciate them. Mathewes asserts, "We must learn how to be joyful, that joy is a capacity that must be developed."[13] To strengthen happiness and wellbeing, we need to be intentional about looking for, experiencing, and appreciating the everyday joyful experiences that come our way.

Gratitude is a joyful emotion, and practices that foster it are among the wisest easy steps we can take to cultivate joy. When used regularly, gratitude practices help us adopt a more positive and appreciative orientation toward the world. We become more aware of the good things and good people in our life. We focus more on the value of what we already have—a home, a good job, loving relationships—rather than trying to acquire more. Dozens of studies show that simple gratitude practices, like the one that follows, enhance our capacities to experience joyful emotions. For example, researchers explored the benefits of daily gratitude among parents of small children.[14] They found that when parents took time at the end of the day to write or reflect on something they were grateful for, they were more satisfied with their daily lives, experienced significantly less stress, and felt closer to their children.

PRACTICING GRATITUDE

This simple practice has been used in dozens of studies, and it consistently evokes joyful emotions. It takes only a few minutes at the end of a day.

Begin by thinking back over the day. Identify three things that you are grateful for. Look for things that made you feel joy in some form, even if it was just a whisper of it. Then, write several sentences that describe why you feel grateful for these things. Including details and rich descriptions will strengthen the beneficial effects of your gratitude. Strive to reach beyond simple statements like "I am grateful for my partner"; be more specific, like "I am grateful for the way my partner took time today to show me how special I am. She surprised me with a sweet text in the middle of the day telling me she was thinking about me, and she wanted to tell me how much love she felt for me. I am so grateful for her, and for the way her text made me feel." Details help deepen your experience of gratitude and are more likely to evoke joy. This practice can be done in as little as ten minutes. If you are not able to write, take time to reflect mentally on what you are grateful for.

Consider sharing these gratitude reflections with another person. This can reinforce and strengthen their beneficial effects and may also evoke joy in them. You might also invite that person to share their gratitude reflections with you. Shared gratitude is also a pathway to joy.

Joy Builds Psychological Resources

Joyful emotions create new psychological resources that are beneficial for wellbeing. They do this by broadening our capacity to think expansively, creatively, and thoughtfully.[15] Joyful emotions foster a more open, curious mindset that increases our capacity to learn, explore, and grow. Studies have demonstrated that after people listened to a favorite song, for example, their visual awareness was significantly enhanced: They literally saw more due to the increased attentional resources that joy created.[16] Other studies show that joyful emotions increase people's creativity, enhance their capacity to make good decisions, and foster a more positive and helpful orientation toward difficult situations.

Over time, learning, insight, creativity, and other broadening effects created by joyful emotions form the foundations we need to build new psychological resources.[17] For example, wonder broadens our capacity to take in new information and experiences while encouraging us to explore; as a result, we gain new knowledge and insights. Serenity heightens our ability to savor the goodness and meaningfulness of life, and builds our capacity to be more open to ways in which we can integrate our values into daily goals and priorities. Inspiration helps us imagine ways to excel and reach toward our personal best, motivating us to strive for personal growth.

These broaden-and-build effects create upward spirals that can enhance and help sustain wellbeing over long periods.[18] Broaden-and-build spirals increase the positive boost we get out of everyday joyful events like helping others, playing a game, reading a good book, and praying. These create the capacity for us to experience more broaden-and-build gains from the use of wise practices such as mindfulness, perspective shifting, growth mindset practices, intentional acts of kindness, and relational practices, among others. These enhanced wise practices then create more joy, leading to a continuing upward spiral.

In turn, these upward spirals also create approach motivation, a close cousin to intrinsic motivation (see chapter nine), which prompts us to take an energized, eager orientation toward goal striving.[19] Approach motivation urges us to work toward valued goals and provides the energy we need to strive with persistence toward them with a positive, optimistic attitude. This motivation can cause us to exceed expectations and go beyond what we previously thought possible. In other words, excellence is often the outcome of approach motivation.

Upward spirals are one of the primary ways that regular use of wise practices can create significant increases in wellbeing. A wise practice helps us address a wellbeing need while creating joyful emotions. Broaden-and-build effects follow and increase our capacity to address the need more intentionally and persistently. As a result, a wise practice has an even stronger effect. This upward spiral continues, and the benefits accumulate over time.

Savoring practices are another wise way to notice and appreciate the joyful experiences in our lives.[20] Like gratitude practices, they can also help fuel upward spirals. Savoring means focusing on and appreciating the goodness of positive experience. It prolongs the joy of these experiences and helps us integrate them into positive memories that we can recall and experience again.

SAVORING

When we savor something, we pay close attention to what is pleasing, enjoyable, tasty, or otherwise good, and we take time to appreciate and relish that goodness. Think about how people taste wine. They swirl it in the glass to appreciate its colors. They smell the wine and identify all of the different aromas as they enjoy its essence. And then, they taste: swishing it around in their mouth, noticing and naming all of the different flavors. This is an example of savoring.

We can take a simpler approach by pausing—even briefly—to focus on a positive experience, to be intentional about noticing and dwelling on what makes it so good. When you take that first bite of dessert, pay attention to the flavors and textures that make it so delicious. Or, when you are watching a favorite movie with someone you love, step back for a moment to appreciate how much you are enjoying that experience.

We can amplify the benefits of savoring by pairing it with a gratitude practice. Shared savoring experiences are also good ways to enhance joy. Talk about what you are enjoying, swap bites of delicious food, hug each other for all of the fun you are having. Express your joy! Laugh, clap, yell—any embodiment of joy is another way to savor it.

Joy Deepens Our Connections with Others

Among the richest sources of joy are our relationships with others and the experiences we share with them. Shared joy can also strengthen our relationships by creating "positivity resonance," which is an upwelling of three experiences: sharing joyful emotions with other people, being psychologically in sync with them, and engaging in verbal and non-verbal expressions of care and concern.[21] It happens in momentary exchanges, like when partners glance lovingly at each other or friends laugh together about an inside joke, and in more extended interactions, like when colleagues work together, parents play with their children, and friends go on vacation together. Positivity resonance happens in situations ranging from calmer and quieter experiences, like cuddling with your partner as you watch TV or reading quietly to a child, to more raucous and energized situations, like attending a rock concert or New Year's Eve party with friends.

Positivity resonance begins when we experience common joyful emotions, laughing at a funny joke, feeling inspired by someone's courage, or that wonderful feeling when we are having a great time with other people. As positivity resonance grows, we experience being in sync or really "clicking" with others. We match each other's emotions, physical movements, facial expressions, and thoughts. The boundaries between ourselves and others become blurred as we feel a sense of oneness or unity with them. Our capacity to understand each other, anticipate each other's needs, and read each other's body language and unspoken communication is enhanced because actual brain-to-brain connections can form between you and other people, known as neural coupling.[22] Brain-scanning studies show that during positivity resonance, the connection between people's brains "is analogous to a wireless communication system in which two brains are coupled via the transmission of a physical signal."[23] When we have a great time with friends at dinner, pray together at church, dance at a wedding reception, hug people when we are reunited, or cheer with fans at a ball game, we are much more in tune because our bodies and brains are synchronized.

During positivity resonance we embody our joy with high fives, hugs, laughter, clapping, and dancing. These gestures convey belonging, affection, care, and love, which evoke more joyful emotions. We offer heartfelt expressions of how much we value other people, and we receive similar expressions from them. These behavioral manifestations also magnify the positive affect we experience by making it more poignant and keenly felt, and more salient and meaningful.

LISTENING

Listening and capitalizing practices from chapter six are wise ways to foster positivity resonance. It feels good to have someone really listen to what we want to say. Whether it is sharing a concern or a piece of really good news, or just talking about everyday events, both the speaker and listener benefit from a good conversation.

Even brief conversations can create positivity resonance. At the gym I look forward to greeting the check-in staff each day. It takes two to three minutes, but I always enjoy making that brief but very human connection. I think of this at stores that have self-checkout lanes. I use them, but realize I am missing an opportunity to create positivity resonance with someone else. A new, wiser practice for me would be to go through the checkout lanes staffed by a person and offer a warm greeting and thanks. It won't take much longer, and it will have the added benefit of creating authentic happiness for at least two people.

> Where are your everyday opportunities to create positivity resonance? Consider selecting one with someone you know, and a second with a more casual acquaintance. While you practice, savor the goodness of making a human connection with someone.

We grow emotionally closer to people during experiences of shared joy. As we experience more positivity with others, we come to trust them more.[24] The frequency of positivity resonance experiences among married and committed couples is a strong predictor of the quality of the relationship and how long it will last. Marriage researcher John Gottman has found that couples who experience more positive interactions are much more likely to have strong, lasting relationships.[25]

Joy Restores and Strengthens Self-Integrity

Contemporary life often subjects us to psychological threats to our sense of self-worth. When we experience personal offenses (someone insults your college or mocks the way you talk) or even minor rude behaviors (someone steps in front of you in the grocery line or does not respond to your cheerful "How are you?"), we often feel that our basic dignity has been impugned. When we can't get through all of the tasks on our to-do lists; when we feel at odds with our spouse, partner, or coworker; or when the pressures to measure up become intense, most of the detrimental effects likely come through the way these experiences undermine our basic sense of "being good enough." More significant events, like receiving negative feedback about something we did, experiencing a financial setback, or losing a job, can be even more damaging to our self-integrity. We take them as evidence of personal deficiencies.

Joyful practices can restore and strengthen self-integrity.[26] They help us affirm an essential goodness that lies at the core of who we are. Prosocial behaviors—helping others, intentional acts of kindness, expressions of gratitude, participating in a volunteer group, holding a door open for someone—can remind us of our positive characteristics and capacities. Spending time with people we love, working with others on high-value projects, and shared STEs can reinforce our connections with the people and things that matter most to us.

Self-affirmation practices strengthen self-integrity, partly by fostering joyful emotions about ourselves. A self-affirmation is an act that demonstrates your adequacy and helps you acknowledge and affirm your basic goodness. Even acts that might seem small can be highly effective in restoring a sense of self-worth. Geoffrey Cohen and David Sherman, the leading researchers of self-affirmations, offer these examples: "A stressed employee who cares for his children or merely reflects on the personal importance of his family; an ill resident of a nursing home who enacts a small measure of control over daily visitations; and a lonely patient who, receiving a personal note from her doctor, realizes that others care for her."[27]

Self-affirmations work by helping us adopt a more expansive view of ourselves. They create a psychological time-out, a chance to step back and regain perspective on who we are and what really matters. When we focus on some aspect of ourselves that we regard as "good," we feel uplifted and hopeful, which in turn engenders a more expansive view of ourselves and our lives. We are less self-critical and more self-accepting. This broader perspective restores our confidence in our ability to overcome difficulties, bolstering our coping skills and increasing our resilience. Because affirmations reinforce our sense of connection to the more important and valuable aspects of life, they also strengthen our sense of meaning and purpose. We are grounded in a positive sense of ourselves, hopeful views of our life, and secure connections to people and things that matter most.

Among the wisest self-affirmation practices are values affirmations. Recall the study from chapter one where, during the first week at a new high school, at-risk students reflected on something important to them. That reflection strengthened their self-integrity, which in turn led to improved academic performance.

VALUES AFFIRMATIONS

Begin by taking time to remind yourself of one of your core values. Take a moment to reflect on it and why it is important to you. Writing a description of that value can help you clarify and crystallize your thoughts and feel how important it is to you. This will help you experience the joyfulness of that value.

Then, recall a time in which you acted on the value. Bring that experience to mind and explore in rich detail the situation, the people present, the things you did, and what was at stake for you during that experience. Allow yourself to feel joyful—proud, inspired, enthusiastic—about your actions. You are not being boastful or immodest, but rather you are affirming an essentially good aspect of who you are. Consider writing about what you are feeling, and perhaps practice emotional granularity to encourage deeper reflections about your innate goodness and stronger experiences of joy.

Studies show that values affirmations like this can restore self-integrity and motivate positive behaviors in a variety of situations. For example, a study of high-body-mass-index women found that those who engaged in a values affirmation practice maintained or reduced their weight over two years, while a control group who did not participate in values affirmations increased their weight.[28] Values affirmations can restore and strengthen willpower and agency, which enhance our capacity to strive successfully toward important goals.[29] Perhaps the most remarkable insight from research is that practicing even once can have lasting benefits.

KEY INSIGHTS

Joyful emotions are the strongest pathway for nourishing and sustaining happiness. Wise practices help you notice and appreciate everyday experiences that are sources of joy.

Joy broadens your capacity to think clearly, constructively, and creatively, and builds new psychological resources that help strengthen and sustain wellbeing.

Shared experiences with important others can be powerful sources of joy that, in turn, strengthen those relationships.

The joy created by values affirmations can restore and strengthen self-integrity, especially when we are exposed to events that undermine our sense of self-worth.

FURTHER READING

How We Heal: Uncover Your Power and Set Yourself Free by Alexandra Elle: A lovely guide for bringing more joy into your life.

Thanks!: How Practicing Gratitude Can Make You Happier by Robert A. Emmons: An accessible exploration of the science of gratitude by a leading wellbeing researcher.

Positivity: Groundbreaking Research to Release Your Inner Optimist and Thrive by Barbara Fredrickson: A deep dive into the science of positive moods and emotions.

Shift: Managing Your Emotions—so They Don't Manage You by Ethan Kross: A fantastic guide to emotions, emotion regulation, and building authentic happiness.

CHAPTER ELEVEN

Wisdom for Journeying Well

I'm often asked questions like "What is the secret to wellbeing?" and "What is one thing everyone should do for their wellbeing?" Those kinds of questions are based upon flawed assumptions that there is one great practice everyone should use or a single insight that will unlock sustained wellbeing. Your path is as unique as you are. Science offers the insights and guidance you need to find and follow the right path, but you have to undertake your own journey.

Like life, your wellbeing journey will have its inevitable ups and downs, and its good, bad, and sometimes ugly surprises. Wellbeing is fundamentally about living well, living a life that you believe is good in the midst of whatever you encounter on that journey. And like life, the journey of wellbeing has to be lived as it unfolds, step-by-step. The old clichés that tell us yesterday is already gone and can't be lived again, and tomorrow is a dream beyond our reach, are very wise. It is the way we live this minute, this hour, this day that matters for our wellbeing. How we live our days is, after all, how we journey through life.

In this final chapter I am going to step a bit beyond the hard scientific evidence and share three of the most important insights I have distilled from more than thirty years of exploring and learning about wellbeing. These insights—be faithful, hopeful, and loving—are my way of summarizing what I believe is essential wisdom for how to nurture and sustain your head, heart, and spirit as you journey forward. Faithfulness grounds you in your values, hope keeps you moving forward during challenges, and love connects you deeply with yourself and others.

Be Faithful

In chapter eight I shared that meaning arises from experiencing purpose, significance, and certitude, and that claiming and living our core values is essential for experiencing meaning. Being faithful expands and deepens our understanding of meaning. Faithfulness is dedication and devotion to your core values, to your spiritual or religious beliefs, and to a way of living that, for you, embodies the highest and best virtues. It goes beyond building your major life priorities and commitments around your core values. Faithfulness is orienting your whole life around these ideals so that you strive each day to enact and embody them.

Faithfulness is "translogical": While rationally, clearly articulated thoughts and careful reasoning are necessary elements of establishing your values, beliefs, and virtues, the commitments and devotions that are essential to faithfulness cannot be fully analyzed, explained, or justified. As philosophers Charles Taylor and Ronald Dworkin point out, we assent to the fundamental importance and truthfulness of our values, beliefs, and virtues.[1] We hold them to be intrinsically higher, incomparable, beyond comparison; because of this, they capture and compel our admiration, respect, and devotion.[2]

Faithfulness is what compels people to work in extremely difficult situations—like many of the humanitarian workers, clergy, and global health workers I studied—and willingly endure ongoing self-sacrifice because of their deep commitment to making the world a better place. I see faithfulness in the lives of people I admire, and perhaps you do as well. Their lives are more deeply oriented around their high ideals. And their commitment to those ideals and their dedication to living them out is the source of the unusual depth, richness, and meaningfulness I see in their lives.

As wise elders throughout time have taught, being faithful is a lifelong endeavor. Dedication and devotion take shape over time, growing stronger as we enact them, day by day. Our capacity to live faithfully unfolds over time, sometimes through important growth experiences or major accomplishments, but much more often through the smaller things we do each day.

Faithfulness requires courage—to resist our darker motivations, to do the hard work of becoming a better person, to live what we value and believe when other people and social pressures push us hard in other directions. It requires the fortitude to keep striving to live out our ideals when the journey of life gets tough or bleak.

Based on my years of study, I think being faithful is the defining characteristic of people who flourish over their lifetime. If there is a "secret" to wellbeing, I think this is it.

Be Hopeful

Václav Havel was a Czechoslovakian statesman, author, and dissident who worked to liberate his homeland from oppression under its Communist regime. He lived through dark and terrible times and was imprisoned multiple times for his political beliefs. Yet he eventually became president of a free Czech Republic. He maintained that it was always hope that gave direction and meaning to his life, sustaining him through his most difficult experiences. "The kind of hope I think about," he wrote,

> especially in situations that are particularly hopeless, such as prison, I understand above all as a state of mind, not a state of the world . . . It is an orientation of the spirit, an orientation of the heart; it transcends the world that is immediately experienced, and is anchored somewhere beyond its horizons. Hope, in this deep and powerful sense, is not the same as joy that things are going well, or willingness to invest in enterprises that are obviously headed for early success, but, rather, an ability to work for something because it is good, not just because it stands a chance to succeed.[3]

Case studies, historical accounts, and personal testimonies of people who have endured extreme hardship show that in times of difficulty, it is hope that sustains them and inspires them to carry on. It nourishes and preserves their sense of meaning even in the darkest of times. "Hope," primate researcher and conservationist Jane Goodall asserted, "is what enables us to keep going in the face of adversity. It is what we desire to happen, but we must be prepared to work hard to make it so."[4] Hope does this because it changes our orientation toward the future. As South African Archbishop Desmond Tutu affirmed, "Hope is being able to see that there is light in the darkness."[5] We see possibilities for making positive change and are inspired to work toward them. And hope opens our eyes to ways we can participate in making that better future a reality; faithfulness to that hope inspires us to work toward that better future. As civil rights activist and member of Congress John Lewis wrote, "I discovered that you have to have this sense of faith that what you're moving toward is already done, the power to believe that you can visualize that sense of your own being toward that day."[6]

We have to find and claim this kind of hope. It's hard to do that when life is whizzing by and the pressures to perform, succeed, and measure up are so strong. Even so, I am convinced that without this kind of hope, we will eventually find ourselves lost on our journey. The hopes you have for your children, your spouse or partner, the work you are doing, and how the world might be a better place are essential nourishment for your heart, your head, and your soul.

Find and remain faithful to hope, and no matter where you are on your journey, no matter how difficult it is, I believe it will sustain you.

Be Loving

The Framingham and Grant studies have definitively established that good relationships in all areas of our life are essential for our wellbeing. While studies have revealed some of the elements of good relationships, this research is limited because, as eminent relationship experts criticize, it has failed to fully explore love. There are many studies of romantic love between intimate partners, but far fewer studies of either companionate love, which forms positive family relationships, friendships, and coworker relationships, or compassionate love, which animates the goodwill, kindness, and respect that create positive interactions with even casual acquaintances. Both companionate and compassionate love are essential for the welfare of individuals and social groups.

The principle of "be loving" emphasizes the importance of prioritizing good relationships even in the briefest of social encounters. The way we treat others influences our own wellbeing as well as theirs.[7] When we are selfish or hurtful to others, we are diminished. We suffer, perhaps in imperceptible ways, but those sufferings accumulate and can significantly undermine our wellbeing. When we are kind to others, when we show respect for them, our wellbeing is strengthened. We are ennobled, often in small but still significant ways, because we have acted well.

One wise way to conceptualize your social ecosystem is as a series of concentric circles. Your intimate partner, closest family relationships, and strongest friendships are in the innermost circle. The first concentric ring includes other family relationships and friendships, perhaps also your connection to a valued coworker, a religious leader, or a mentor. As you move outward, the relationships become more distant, superficial, and casual. Being loving encourages you to pull people closer to the middle and expand the sizes of the inner rings. Given that every single interaction matters, even transitory interactions should be approached with kindness, respectfulness, and care. You never journey alone.

Your Wellbeing, Your Journey

You may have surmised that these three insights are expressions of three of my core values. They are also aspirations that guide me in my journey. A few years ago I gave up my tenured position at Notre Dame because following these aspirations meant I needed to journey into new territory. I needed to leave my comfortable post in academia to be faithful to those values, and also to follow my hope that I could find new and better ways to help people. This book is one gesture of that hope.

Where will you go next on your journey? Step back and plan your next destination. What wise practices will you bring into your daily life? Step easy so the benefits of wise practices will add up over time to strengthen your wellbeing. Who will you invite to journey with you? Step together with someone who will encourage and support you, and whom you can love and care for. As you move forward, ask how faithfulness, hope, and love will shape your journey.

You are ready to go. I wish you the very best on your journey.

Acknowledgments

My deepest thanks to all the people who participated in my research projects. I am especially grateful for those who traveled with me to remote outposts and those who shared their sacred stories with me. Catholic Relief Services was a generous partner, and I am grateful for the time I spent with its amazing staff.

Kevin Hartigan created opportunities for me that changed my research and changed my life. Matt McGarry has been a source of enthusiasm and insight for many years. Thank you, my friends.

Manuela Casti-Yeagley, Sarah Klinedinst, Judy Miller, and Laura Schmucker were the heart of my research team. Thank you for the fun, your hard work, and caring about me and our research.

John Nagy: Thank you for your support and encouragement. Your example of skillful writing helped me immensely.

My thanks to the Lilly Endowment and Templeton Religion Trust for the generous financial support of my research. Special thanks to Craig Dykstra and Chris Coble of Lilly, and Chris Stewart of TRT: You made this book possible.

Dominic Brewer, Dan Cable, Amy Colbert, Mike Crant, Rob Easley, Ira Harris, and John Michel have been colleagues during some of the most important times in my academic career. You were friends when I really needed one.

To the many students I had the privilege of teaching at Mendoza: You are what make Notre Dame so special to me.

Michael McGregor, my writing coach: Thank you for teaching me so much about the craft of writing, and most of all, for helping me finally claim, "I am a writer!"

Laurie Abkemeier, my agent, publishing coach, and advocate: Thank you for taking on a new author. I am deeply grateful for your kindness, wisdom, and guidance.

Leah Wilson, my editor at BenBella, and Clara Tamez, her able assistant: Your gentle guidance taught me so much about writing and made this book much better. Thanks to James Fraleigh for your meticulous copyediting. And to the entire BenBella team: You have been a dream to work with.

My friends in Lost River: Dan Fitz, Steve Marker, Joe Polumbo, and John Rosato. I miss hanging out with you guys! Know that I cherish your friendship.

Michael Milano: You are my *anam cara*. Thank you for many years of friendship.

My parents, Mary and Chuck, have been among my most ardent champions. Their wisdom and love have been constant sources of strength all of my life. Mom: I miss our conversations and your warm hugs. Dad: You are *my* rock. My brother, Steve, believed I could write this book long before I did. Steve: Thanks for your enthusiasm and enduring support.

Keaton and Maíra: Your love and affection have lifted me more times than you know. Mateo and Leo: You are my joy boys! I love each of you deeply. The times Kim and I spend with you are among our most cherished moments.

Nicholas: I miss you.

Kim: Your love is the constant in my life. You have supported me through so much. No thanks is sufficient for all you have done, no words can convey how much you mean to me. IHA2.

Notes

Chapter 1

1. The Harris Poll, "Mental Health: A Comprehensive Look at Harris Poll Research," May 12, 2023, https://www.theharrispoll.com/briefs/mental-health-a-comprehensive-look-at-harris-poll-research/.
2. Cigna Healthcare, *Cigna Healthcare 360 Global Well-Being Survey*, accessed November 25, 2025.
3. Gregory M. Walton and Timothy D. Wilson, "Wise Interventions: Psychological Remedies for Social and Personal Problems," *Psychological Review* 125 (2018): 617–55.
4. Pam A. Mueller and Daniel M. Oppenheimer, "The Pen Is Mightier Than the Keyboard: Advantages of Longhand Over Laptop Note Taking," *Psychological Science* 25 (2014): 1159–68; F. R. Van der Weel and Audrey L. H. Van der Meer, "Handwriting but Not Typewriting Leads to Widespread Brain Connectivity: A High-Density EEG Study with Implications for the Classroom," *Frontiers in Psychology* 14 (2023): 1219945.
5. Sarah A. Hayes-Skelton et al., "A Randomized Clinical Trial Comparing an Acceptance-Based Behavior Therapy to Applied Relaxation for Generalized Anxiety Disorder," *Journal of Consulting and Clinical Psychology* 81 (2013): 761–73; Shelley Viskovich and Kenneth I.

Pakenham, "Pilot Evaluation of a Web-Based Acceptance and Commitment Therapy Program to Promote Mental Health Skills in University Students," *Journal of Clinical Psychology* 74 (2018): 2047–69.

6. David S. Yeager et al., "A National Experiment Reveals Where a Growth Mindset Improves Achievement," *Nature* 573 (2019): 364–69.
7. David K. Sherman et al., "Deflecting the Trajectory and Changing the Narrative: How Self-Affirmation Affects Academic Performance and Motivation Under Identity Threat," *Journal of Personality and Social Psychology* 104 (2013): 591–618; Geoffrey L. Cohen et al., "Recursive Processes in Self-Affirmation: Intervening to Close the Minority Achievement Gap," *Science* 324 (2009): 400–403.
8. Connie W. Tsao and Ramachandran S. Vasan, "The Framingham Heart Study: Past, Present and Future," *International Journal of Epidemiology* 44 (2015): 1763–66.
9. Nicholas A. Christakis and James H. Fowler, *Connected: The Surprising Power of Our Social Networks and How They Shape Our Lives* (Little, Brown, 2009).
10. Christakis, *Connected*, 110.
11. Nina Wirtz et al., "What About the Leader? Crossover of Emotional Exhaustion and Work Engagement from Followers to Leaders," *Journal of Occupational Health Psychology* 22 (2017): 86–97.
12. Chloé Meredith et al., "'Burnout Contagion' Among Teachers: A Social Network Approach," *Journal of Occupational and Organizational Psychology* 93 (2020): 328–52.
13. Adam D. I. Kramer et al., "Experimental Evidence of Massive-Scale Emotional Contagion Through Social Networks," *Proceedings of the National Academy of Sciences* 111 (2014): 8788–90.
14. Michael G. Wheaton et al., "Is Fear of COVID-19 Contagious? The Effects of Emotion Contagion and Social Media Use on Anxiety in Response to the Coronavirus Pandemic," *Frontiers in Psychology* 11 (2021): 567379.

Chapter 2

1. Darrin M. McMahon, *Happiness: A History* (Atlantic Monthly Press, 2006).
2. Darrin M. McMahon, "The Ideal of Happiness," *Social Research* 77 (2010): 469–90.
3. William James, *The Varieties of Religious Experience* (Modern Library, 1902), 78.
4. Ruth Whippman, *America the Anxious: How Our Pursuit of Happiness Is Creating a Nation of Nervous Wrecks* (St. Martin's Press, 2016).
5. Barbara Ehrenreich, *Bright-Sided: How the Relentless Promotion of Positive Thinking Has Undermined America* (Metropolitan Books, 2009).
6. John F. Helliwell et al., eds., *World Happiness Report 2024*, Wellbeing Research Centre, accessed August 5, 2024, https://www.worldhappiness.report.
7. Barbara Fredrickson, "Updated Thinking on Positivity Ratios," *American Psychologist* 68 (2013): 814–22; Robert M. Schwartz and James Grice, "Positive Ratios Revisited: Reports of the Theory's Death Have Been Greatly Exaggerated," *The Journal of Positive Psychology* 17 (2022): 1–9.
8. Sonja Lyubomirsky et al., "The Benefits of Frequent Positive Affect: Does Happiness Lead to Success?" *Psychological Bulletin* 131 (2005): 803–55.
9. Sarah D. Pressman and Sheldon Cohen, "Does Positive Affect Influence Health?" *Psychological Bulletin* 131 (2005): 925–71.
10. Sheldon Cohen et al., "Ten Surprising Facts About Stressful Life Events and Disease Risk," *Annual Review of Psychology* 70 (2019): 577–97.
11. Roy F. Baumeister and John Tierney, *Willpower: Rediscovering the Greatest Human Strength* (Penguin Press, 2011); Stevan E. Hobfoll et al., "Expanding the Science of Resilience: Conserving

Resources in the Aid of Adaptation," *Psychological Inquiry* 26 (2015): 174–80.

12. Geoffrey L. Cohen and David K. Sherman, "The Psychology of Change: Self-Affirmation and Social Psychological Intervention," *Annual Review of Psychology* 65 (2014): 333–71.
13. Susan T. Fiske, "Envy Up, Scorn Down: How Comparison Divides Us," *American Psychologist* 65 (2010): 698–706.
14. Julianne Holt-Lunstad, ed., *Our Epidemic of Loneliness and Isolation: The U.S. Surgeon General's Advisory on the Healing Effects of Social Connection and Community* (Office of the US Surgeon General, 2023, 23).
15. Vivek H. Murthy, *Together: Loneliness, Health and What Happens When We Find Connection* (Profile Books, 2021).
16. Brooke C. Feeney and Nancy L. Collins, "A New Look at Social Support: A Theoretical Perspective on Thriving Through Relationships," *Personality and Social Psychology Review* 19 (2015): 113–47.
17. Crystal L. Park, "Making Sense of the Meaning Literature: An Integrative Review of Meaning Making and Its Effects on Adjustment to Stressful Life Events," *Psychological Bulletin* 136 (2010): 257–301.
18. Jeffrey A. Hanson and Tyler J. VanderWeele, "The Comprehensive Measure of Meaning: Psychological and Philosophical Foundations," in *Measuring Well-Being*, ed. Mathew T. Lee et al. (Oxford University Press, 2021).
19. Harold G. Koenig, *Religion and Mental Health: Research and Clinical Applications* (Academic Press, 2018).
20. Frank Martela and Michael F. Steger, "The Role of Significance Relative to the Other Dimensions of Meaning in Life—an Examination Utilizing the Three Dimensional Meaning in Life Scale," *The Journal of Positive Psychology* 18 (2023): 606–26.
21. Susan R. Wolf and John Koethe, *Meaning in Life and Why It Matters* (Princeton University Press, 2010).

22. Lisa Miller, *The Awakened Brain: The New Science of Spirituality and Our Quest for an Inspired Life* (Random House, 2021).
23. Kenneth I. Pargament, ed., *APA Handbook of Psychology, Religion, and Spirituality* (American Psychological Association, 2013).

Chapter 3

1. Robert M. Sapolsky, *Why Zebras Don't Get Ulcers: An Updated Guide to Stress, Stress-Related Diseases, and Coping* (W. H. Freeman, 1998), 20.
2. Belden C. Lane, *Backpacking with the Saints: Wilderness Hiking as Spiritual Practice* (Oxford University Press, 2015), xvii.
3. Janice K. Kiecolt-Glaser et al., "Stress Reactivity: What Pushes Us Higher, Faster, and Longer—and Why It Matters," *Current Directions in Psychological Science* 29 (2020): 492–98.
4. Mark Brackett, *Permission to Feel: Unlocking the Power of Emotions to Help Our Kids, Ourselves, and Our Society Thrive* (Celadon Books, 2019), 17.
5. Elissa Epel, *The Stress Prescription: Seven Days to More Joy and Ease* (Penguin, 2022), 20.
6. Robert M. Sapolsky, *Why Zebras Don't Get Ulcers: An Updated Guide to Stress, Stress-Related Diseases, and Coping* (St. Martin's Griffin, 2004), 207, Kindle.
7. Shian-Ling Keng et al., "Effects of Mindfulness on Psychological Health: A Review of Empirical Studies," *Clinical Psychology Review* 31 (2011): 1041–56.
8. Eyal Ophir et al., "Cognitive Control in Media Multitaskers," *Proceedings of the National Academy of Sciences* 106 (2009): 15583–87.
9. Daniel Goleman and Richard J. Davidson, *Altered Traits: Science Reveals How Meditation Changes Your Mind, Brain, and Body* (Avery, 2017); Yi-Yuan Tang et al., "The Neuroscience of Mindfulness Meditation," *Nature Reviews Neuroscience* 16 (2015): 213–25.

10. Jenny Gu et al., "How Do Mindfulness-Based Cognitive Therapy and Mindfulness-Based Stress Reduction Improve Mental Health and Wellbeing? A Systematic Review and Meta-Analysis of Mediation Studies," *Clinical Psychology Review* 37 (2015): 1–12.
11. Alexandra D. Crosswell et al., "Deep Rest: An Integrative Model of How Contemplative Practices Combat Stress and Enhance the Body's Restorative Capacity," *Psychological Review* 131 (2024): 247–70.
12. Amit Bernstein et al., "Metacognitive Processes Model of Decentering: Emerging Methods and Insights," *Current Opinion in Psychology* 28 (2019): 245–51.
13. David R. Vago and Fadel Zeidan, "The Brain on Silent: Mind Wandering, Mindful Awareness, and States of Mental Tranquility," *Annals of the New York Academy of Sciences* 1373 (2016): 96–113.
14. Richard W. Levenson, Paul Ekman and Mathieu Ricard. "Meditation and the Startle Response: A Case Study." *Emotion* 12 (2012): 650-8.

Chapter 4

1. Ethan Kross, *Chatter: The Voice in Our Heads, Why It Matters, and How to Harness It* (Crown, 2021), 17.
2. Bessel van der Kolk, *The Body Keeps the Score: Brain, Mind, and Body in the Healing of Trauma* (Penguin, 2014), 21.
3. American Institute of Stress, "Worrying Workplace Stress Statistics," *AIS Daily Life Blog*, last modified September 25, 2019, https://www.stress.org/42-worrying-workplace-stress-statistics (site discontinued).
4. American Psychological Association, "Stress in America 2024: A Nation in Political Turmoil," last modified October 25, 2024, https://www.apa.org/pubs/reports/stress-in-america/2024/2024-stress-in-america-full-report.pdf.
5. American College Health Association, "2023 Well-Being Assessment," accessed January 2, 2024, https://www.acha.org/wp-content/uploads

/2024/07/ACHA_WELL-BEING_ASSESSMENT_FALL_2023_REFERENCE_GROUP_DATA_REPORT.pdf.

6. Steven C. Hayes et al., "Open, Aware, and Active: Contextual Approaches as an Emerging Trend in the Behavioral and Cognitive Therapies," *Annual Review of Clinical Psychology* 7 (2011): 141–68; Society for Human Resource Management, "The State of Employee Mental Health in 2024," April 30, 2024, https://www.shrm.org/topics-tools/news/inclusion-diversity/burnout-shrm-research-2024.
7. Sally Winston and Martin N. Seif, *Overcoming Unwanted Intrusive Thoughts: A CBT-Based Guide to Getting over Frightening, Obsessive, or Disturbing Thoughts* (New Harbinger Publications, 2017), 6.
8. Kross, *Chatter*, 47.
9. Brett Q. Ford et al., "The Psychological Health Benefits of Accepting Negative Emotions and Thoughts: Laboratory, Diary, and Longitudinal Evidence," *Journal of Personality and Social Psychology* 115 (2018): 1075–92.
10. Elissa Epel, *The Stress Prescription: Seven Days to More Joy and Ease* (Penguin, 2022), 66.
11. Epel, *The Stress Prescription*, 66.
12. Vera U. Ludwig et al., "Self-Regulation Without Force: Can Awareness Leverage Reward to Drive Behavior Change?" *Perspectives on Psychological Science* 15 (2020): 1382–99.
13. Kross, *Chatter*, 66.
14. Brian E. Wisco et al., "Self-Distancing from Trauma Memories Reduces Physiological but Not Subjective Emotional Reactivity Among Veterans with Posttraumatic Stress Disorder," *Clinical Psychological Science* 3 (2015): 956–63.
15. Shana Cole et al., "Out of Reach and Under Control: Distancing as a Self-Control Strategy," *Personality and Social Psychology Bulletin* 47 (2020): 939–52.

16. Lisa Feldman Barrett, *How Emotions Are Made: The Secret Life of the Brain* (Houghton Mifflin Harcourt, 2017).
17. Ford, "The Psychological Health Benefits of Accepting Negative Emotions and Thoughts."
18. Daniel Kahneman, *Thinking, Fast and Slow* (Farrar, Straus and Giroux, 2013).
19. Lauren A. M. Lebois et al., "Augmentation of Extinction and Inhibitory Learning in Anxiety and Trauma-Related Disorders," *Annual Review of Clinical Psychology* 15 (2019): 257–84.
20. Adam Grant, *Think Again: The Power of Knowing What You Don't Know* (Viking, 2021).
21. Grant, *Think Again,* 11.
22. Vicki S. Helgeson et al., "A Meta-Analytic Review of Benefit Finding and Growth," *Journal of Consulting and Clinical Psychology* 74 (2006): 797–816.
23. Kyla Rankin and Kate Sweeny, "Preparing Silver Linings for a Cloudy Day: The Consequences of Preemptive Benefit Finding," *Personality and Social Psychology Bulletin* 48 (2021): 1255–68.
24. Veronika Brandstätter and Katharina Bernecker, "Persistence and Disengagement in Personal Goal Pursuit," *Annual Review of Psychology* 73 (2022): 271–99; Wendy Wood, "Habits, Goals, and Effective Behavior Change," *Current Directions in Psychological Science* 33 (2024): 226–32.
25. Wendy Wood, *Good Habits, Bad Habits: The Science of Making Positive Changes That Stick* (Farrar, Straus and Giroux, 2019), 17.
26. Brian Wansink and Collin R. Payne, "Eating Behavior and Obesity at Chinese Buffets," *Obesity* 16 (2008): 1957–60.
27. Wood, *Good Habits,* 30.
28. Sabine Sonnentag et al., "Recovery from Work: Advancing the Field Toward the Future," *Annual Review of Organizational Psychology and Organizational Behavior* 9 (2022): 33–60.

Chapter 5

1. Tait D. Shanafelt et al., "Changes in Burnout and Satisfaction with Work–Life Integration in Physicians and the General US Working Population Between 2011 and 2017," *Mayo Clinic Proceedings* 94 (2019): 1–14.
2. Tait D. Shanafelt et al., "Changes in Burnout and Satisfaction with Work–Life Integration in Physicians and the General US Working Population Between 2011 and 2023," *Mayo Clinic Proceedings* 100 (2024): 1142–58.
3. Amelia Aldao et al., "Emotion-Regulation Strategies Across Psychopathology: A Meta-Analytic Review," *Clinical Psychology Review* 30 (2010): 217–37.
4. Roy F. Baumeister et al., *Losing Control: How and Why People Fail at Self-Regulation* (Academic Press, 1994).
5. Wilken Wehrt et al., "More than a Muscle: How Self-Control Motivation, Depletion, and Self-Regulation Strategies Impact Task Performance," *Journal of Organizational Behavior* 43 (2020): 1358–76.
6. George A. Bonanno, *The End of Trauma: How the New Science of Resilience Is Changing How We Think About PTSD* (Basic Books, 2021), 145.
7. Bonanno, *The End of Trauma*, 146.
8. Alia J. Crum et al., "Evaluation of the 'Rethink Stress' Mindset Intervention: A Metacognitive Approach to Changing Mindsets," *Journal of Experimental Psychology: General* 152 (2023): 2603–22.
9. Crum, "Evaluation of the 'Rethink Stress' Mindset Intervention," 2608.
10. Ethan Kross et al., "Self-Talk as a Regulatory Mechanism: How You Do It Matters," *Journal of Personality and Social Psychology* 106 (2014): 304–24.

11. Kristin Naragon-Gainey et al., "The Structure of Common Emotion Regulation Strategies: A Meta-Analytic Examination," *Psychological Bulletin* 143 (2017): 384–427.

12. James W. Pennebaker and John F. Evans, *Expressive Writing: Words That Heal* (Idyll Arbor, 2014).

Chapter 6

1. William T. Grant Foundation, "History," accessed March 17, 2025, https://www.wtgrantfoundation.org/about/history.
2. William T. Grant Foundation, "History."
3. Ken Fuchsman, "Harvard Grant Study of Adult Development: 1938–2022," *Journal of Psychohistory* 51 (2023): 27–44.
4. Robert Waldinger and Marc Schulz, "The Lifelong Power of Close Relationships," *The Wall Street Journal*, January 13, 2023, https://www.wsj.com/articles/the-lifelong-power-of-close-relationships-11673625450.
5. Jeffry A. Simpson and Lorne Campbell, eds., *The Oxford Handbook of Close Relationships* (Oxford University Press, 2013).
6. Robert Waldinger and Marc Schulz, *The Good Life: Lessons from the World's Longest Scientific Study of Happiness* (Simon & Schuster, 2023).
7. Waldinger and Schulz, *The Good Life*, 82.
8. Monique M. H. Pollmann and Catrin Finkenauer, "Investigating the Role of Two Types of Understanding in Relationship Well-Being: Understanding Is More Important Than Knowledge," *Personality and Social Psychology Bulletin* 35 (2009): 1512–27.
9. Kipling D. Williams, "Ostracism," *Annual Review of Psychology* 58 (2007): 425–52.
10. Amy C. Edmondson and Derrick P. Bransby, "Psychological Safety Comes of Age: Observed Themes in an Established Literature," *Annual*

Review of Organizational Psychology and Organizational Behavior 10 (2023): 55–78.

11. Roy F. Baumeister and Mark R. Leary, "The Need to Belong: Desire for Interpersonal Attachments as a Fundamental Human Motivation," *Psychological Bulletin* 117 (1995): 497–529.
12. Margaret S. Clark and Judson R. Mill, "A Theory of Communal (and Exchange) Relationships," in *Handbook of Theories of Social Psychology*, ed. Paul A. M. Van Lange et al., vol. 2 (Sage, 2012).
13. Barbara Fredrickson, *Love 2.0: Creating Happiness and Health in Moments of Connection* (Plume, 2013), 4.
14. Brooke C. Feeney and Nancy L. Collins, "A New Look at Social Support," *Personality and Social Psychology Review* 19 (2015): 113–47.
15. Erica J. Boothby and Margaret S. Clark, "Side by Side: How Merely Being with a Close Other Can Enhance Well-Being," in *Positive Psychology: Established and Emerging Issues*, ed. Dana S. Dunn (Routledge, 2018).
16. Jamil Zaki, "Empathy: A Motivated Account," *Psychological Bulletin* 140 (2014): 1608–47.
17. P. Matthijs Bal et al., "The Influence of Fictional Narrative Experience on Work Outcomes: A Conceptual Analysis and Research Model," *Review of General Psychology* 15 (2011): 361–70.
18. Guy Itzchakov et al., "Listening to Understand: The Role of High-Quality Listening on Speakers' Attitude Depolarization During Disagreements," *Journal of Personality and Social Psychology* 126 (2024): 213–39.
19. Guy Itzchakov and Avraham N. Kluger, "The Listening Circle: A Simple Tool to Enhance Listening and Reduce Extremism Among Employees," *Organizational Dynamics* 46 (2017): 220–26.
20. Shelly L. Gable and Harry T. Reis, "Good News! Capitalizing on Positive Events in an Interpersonal Context," *Advances in Experimental Social Psychology* 42 (2010): 195–257.

21. Brett K. Jakubiak et al., "Affectionate Touch Promotes Shared Positive Activities," *Personality and Social Psychology Bulletin* 49 (2022): 939–54.

22. Brett K. Jakubiak and Brooke C. Feeney, "Hand-in-Hand Combat: Affectionate Touch Promotes Relational Well-Being and Buffers Stress During Conflict," *Personality and Social Psychology Bulletin* 45 (2018): 431–46.

23. Harry T. Reis and Shelly L. Gable, "Responsiveness," *Current Opinion in Psychology* 1 (2015): 67–71.

24. Anita L Vangelisti and Daniel Perlman, *The Cambridge Handbook of Personal Relationships*, 2nd ed. (Cambridge University Press, 2018).

25. Caryl E. Rusbult et al., "'The Part of Me That You Bring Out': Ideal Similarity and the Michelangelo Phenomenon," *Journal of Personality and Social Psychology* 96 (2009): 61–82.

26. Eli J. Finkel, "Complementing the Sculpting Metaphor: Reflections on How Relationship Partners Elicit the Best or the Worst in Each Other," *Review of General Psychology* 23 (2018): 127–32.

27. Amy Canevello and Jennifer Crocker, "Creating Good Relationships: Responsiveness, Relationship Quality, and Interpersonal Goals," *Journal of Personality and Social Psychology* 99 (2010): 78–106.

28. Alixandra Barasch, "The Consequences of Sharing," *Current Opinion in Psychology* 31 (2020): 61–66.

29. Michael L. Slepian and Edythe Moulton-Tetlock, "Confiding Secrets and Well-Being," *Social Psychological and Personality Science* 10 (2019): 472–84.

30. Arthur Aron et al., "The Experimental Generation of Interpersonal Closeness: A Procedure and Some Preliminary Findings," *Personality and Social Psychology Bulletin* 23 (1997): 363–77.

31. Michael E. McCullough et al., "Interpersonal Forgiving in Close Relationships," *Journal of Personality and Social Psychology* 73 (1997): 321–36.

32. Edward P. Lemay and Margaret S. Clark, "How the Head Liberates the Heart: Projection of Communal Responsiveness Guides Relationship Promotion," *Journal of Personality and Social Psychology* 94 (2008): 647–71.
33. Adam Grant, *Give and Take: A Revolutionary Approach to Success* (Viking, 2013), 17.

Chapter 7

1. Delores F. Brisbon, *A Privileged Life: Remembering My Journey* (CreateSpace, 2010), 32.
2. Delores F. Brisbon, *A Privileged Life II: Wisdom from My Journey* (Zion Publishing Services, 2019), 66.
3. Brisbon, *A Privileged Life II*, 67.
4. Cited in Jacqui Banaszynski, "Stories Matter," in *Telling True Stories: A Nonfiction Writers' Guide*, ed. Mark Kramer and Wendy Call (Plumel, 2007), 4.
5. Tilman Habermas and Susan Bluck, "Getting a Life: The Emergence of the Life Story in Adolescence," *Psychological Bulletin* 126 (2000): 748–69.
6. Michael H. Kernis and Brian M. Goldman, "A Multicomponent Conceptualization of Authenticity: Theory and Research," *Advances in Experimental Social Psychology* 38 (2006): 283–357.
7. Tasha Eurich, *Insight: Why We're Not as Self-Aware as We Think, and How Seeing Ourselves Clearly Helps Us Succeed at Work and in Life* (Crown Business, 2017).
8. Susan Sontag and David Rieff, *Reborn: Journals and Notebooks, 1947–1963* (Farrar, Straus and Giroux, 2008), 28.
9. F. R. van der Weel and Audrey F. H. van der Meer, "Handwriting but Not Typewriting Leads to Widespread Brain Connectivity: A

High-Density EEG Study with Implications for the Classroom," *Frontiers in Psychology* 14 (2023): 1219945.

10. Eurich, *Insight.*
11. William James, *The Will to Believe and Other Essays in Popular Philosophy* (Longmans, Green, and Co., 1912).
12. Christopher Peterson and Martin E. P. Seligman, *Character Strengths and Virtues: A Handbook and Classification* (American Psychological Association, 2004).
13. Klodiana Lanaj et al., "Energizing Leaders via Self-Reflection: A Within-Person Field Experiment," *Journal of Applied Psychology* 104 (2019): 1–18.
14. Wiebke Bleidorn et al., "The Policy Relevance of Personality Traits," *The American Psychologist* 74 (2019): 1056–67.
15. Michael C. Ashton and Kibeom Lee, "Age Trends in HEXACO-PI-R Self-Reports," *Journal of Research in Personality* 64 (2016): 102–11.
16. Laura M. Roberts et al. "Composing the Reflected Best-Self Portrait: Building Pathways for Becoming Extraordinary in Work Organizations," *Academy of Management Review* 30 (2013): 712–36.
17. Carl G. Jung, Gerhard Adler, and R. F. C. Hull, *Collected Works of C.G. Jung,* vol. 16 (Princeton University Press, 2014), para. 470.
18. Forrest Hanson, host, "Linking: The Secret to Rewiring Painful Memories," *Being Well* (podcast), April 7, 2025, https://www.rickhanson.com/being-well-podcast-linking-the-secret-to-rewiring-painful-memories.
19. Kristin Neff, *Self-Compassion: The Proven Power of Being Kind to Yourself* (William Morrow, 2011).
20. Kristin D. Neff, "Self-Compassion: Theory, Method, Research, and Intervention," *Annual Review of Psychology* 74 (2023): 193–218.
21. Jack J. Bauer, *The Transformative Self: Personal Growth, Narrative Identity, and the Good Life* (Oxford Academic, 2021).

22. Dan P. McAdams, "The Life Story Interview–II," revised 2007, accessed December 10, 2025, tiny.cc/LifeNarrative.
23. Barack Obama, *Dreams from My Father: A Story of Race and Inheritance* (Random House, 1995).
24. Obama, *Dreams from My Father*, 82.
25. David Remnick, *The Bridge: The Life and Rise of Barack Obama* (Vintage, 2011), 114.
26. Remnick, *The Bridge,* 114.

Chapter 8

1. Lilach Sagiv and Shalom H. Schwartz, "Personal Values Across Cultures," *Annual Review of Psychology* 73 (2022): 517–46.
2. Gordon W. Allport, *The Individual and His Religion: A Psychological Interpretation* (Macmillan, 1950).
3. Brad Stulberg, *Master of Change: How to Excel When Everything Is Changing—Including You* (HarperOne, 2023), 76.
4. Viktor E. Frankl, *Man's Search for Meaning* (Beacon Press, 2006), 105.
5. Edward L. Deci and Richard M. Ryan, "The 'What' and 'Why' of Goal Pursuits: Human Needs and the Self-Determination of Behavior," *Psychological Inquiry* 11 (2000): 227–68.
6. Tim Kasser, "Materialistic Values and Goals," *Annual Review of Psychology* 67 (2016): 489–514.
7. Emma L. Bradshaw et al., "A Meta-Analysis of the Dark Side of the American Dream: Evidence for the Universal Wellness Costs of Prioritizing Extrinsic over Intrinsic Goals," *Journal of Personality and Social Psychology* 124 (2023): 873–99.
8. For reviews of this research see Deci, "The 'What' and 'Why' of Goal Pursuits"; Richard M. Ryan et al., "We Know This Much Is (Meta-Analytically) True: A Meta-Review of Meta-Analytic Findings Evaluating Self-Determination Theory," *Psychological Bulletin* 148 (2022):

813–42; Richard M. Ryan, *The Oxford Handbook of Self-Determination Theory* (Oxford University Press, 2023).

9. Harold G. Koenig et al., *Handbook of Religion and Health*, 3rd ed. (Oxford University Press, 2023).
10. Michael Prinzing et al., "More Than a Momentary Blip in the Universe? Investigating the Link Between Religiousness and Perceived Meaning in Life," *Personality and Social Psychology Bulletin* 49 (2021): 180–96.
11. Gerald Echterhoff et al., "Shared Reality: Experiencing Commonality with Others' Inner States About the World," *Perspectives on Psychological Science* 4 (2009): 496–521.
12. Constantine Sedikides et al., "To Nostalgize: Mixing Memory with Affect and Desire," *Advances in Experimental Social Psychology* 51 (2015): 189–273.
13. Wing-Yee Cheung et al., "Back to the Future: Nostalgia Increases Optimism," *Personality and Social Psychology Bulletin* 39 (2013): 1484–96.
14. Andrew A. Abeyta and Simran Pillarisetty, "Nostalgia Supports a Meaningful Life," *Current Opinion in Psychology* 49 (2023): 101520; David B. Newman et al., "Nostalgia and Well-Being in Daily Life: An Ecological Validity Perspective," *Journal of Personality and Social Psychology* 118 (2020): 325–47.
15. Mark C. Bolino and Adam M. Grant, "The Bright Side of Being Prosocial at Work, and the Dark Side, Too: A Review and Agenda for Research on Other-Oriented Motives, Behavior, and Impact in Organizations," *Academy of Management Annals* 10 (2016): 599–670.
16. Stephen G. Post, ed., *Altruism and Health: Perspectives from Empirical Research* (Oxford Academic, 2007).
17. Bryant P. H. Hui et al., "Rewards of Kindness? A Meta-Analysis of the Link Between Prosociality and Well-Being," *Psychological Bulletin* 146 (2020): 1084–1116.
18. Lisa Miller, *The Awakened Brain: The New Science of Spirituality and Our Quest for an Inspired Life* (Random House, 2021).

19. David Bryce Yaden et al., "The Varieties of Self-Transcendent Experience," *Review of General Psychology* 21 (2017): 143–60.
20. Ian McGregor et al., "Higher Power Dynamics: How Meaning Search and Self-Transcendence Inspire Approach Motivation and Magnanimity," *Journal of Experimental Social Psychology* 102 (2022): 1–17.
21. Dacher Keltner, *Awe: The New Science of Everyday Wonder and How It Can Transform Your Life* (Penguin Press, 2023), 28.
22. Elias C. Acevedo and Jeremy Tost, "Self-Transcendent Experience and Prosociality: Connecting Dispositional Awe, Compassion, and the Moral Foundations," *Personality and Individual Differences* 214 (2023): 1–6.
23. Yang Bai et al., "Awe, Daily Stress, and Elevated Life Satisfaction," *Journal of Personality and Social Psychology* 120 (2021): 837–60.
24. Samantha Hajna et al., "Associations Between Residential Greenspace Exposure and Mortality in 4 645 581 Adults Living in London, UK: A Longitudinal Study," *The Lancet Planetary Health* 7 (2023): e459–68.
25. Rebecca S. Geary et al., "Ambient Greenness, Access to Local Green Spaces, and Subsequent Mental Health: A 10-Year Longitudinal Dynamic Panel Study of 2·3 Million Adults in Wales," *The Lancet Planetary Health* 7 (2023): e809–18.
26. Rico Pohling and Rhett Diessner, "Moral Elevation and Moral Beauty: A Review of the Empirical Literature," *Review of General Psychology* 20 (2016): 412–25.
27. See for example Andrew L. Thomson and Jason T. Siegel, "Elevation: A Review of Scholarship on a Moral and Other-Praising Emotion," *The Journal of Positive Psychology* 12 (2017): 628–38; Dacher Keltner and Eftychia Stamkou, "Possible Worlds Theory: How the Imagination Transcends and Recreates Reality," *Annual Review of Psychology* 76 (2025): 329–58.

Chapter 9

1. Annie Dillard, *The Writing Life* (Harper & Row, 1989).
2. Cal Newport, *Slow Productivity: The Lost Art of Accomplishment Without Burnout* (Portfolio, 2024), 216, 12.
3. Cameron Crowe, "Jerry Maguire Mission Statement," The Uncool, April 25, 2016, http://www.theuncool.com/2016/04/25/jerry-maguire-mission-statement/.
4. Michelle Z. Yang et al., "Evidence That Mental Contrasting Reduces Health Information Avoidance," *Annals of Behavioral Medicine* 57 (2023): 687–92.
5. Newport, *Slow Productivity*, 219.
6. Carol S. Dweck, *Mindset: The New Psychology of Success* (Ballantine Books, 2016).
7. Jeni L. Burnette et al., "Mind-Sets Matter: A Meta-Analytic Review of Implicit Theories and Self-Regulation," *Psychological Bulletin* 139 (2013): 655–701.
8. Jessica Schleider et al., "Implicit Theories and Youth Mental Health Problems: A Random-Effects Meta-Analysis," *Clinical Psychology Review* 35 (2015): 1–9.
9. Michael Norton, *The Ritual Effect: From Habit to Ritual, Harness the Surprising Power of Everyday Actions* (Scribner, 2024).
10. Nicholas M. Hobson et al., "The Psychology of Rituals: An Integrative Review and Process-Based Framework," *Personality and Social Psychology Review* 22 (2018): 260–84.
11. Parker J. Palmer, *The Courage to Teach: Exploring the Inner Landscape of a Teacher's Life* (Jossey-Bass, 1990); Parker J. Palmer, "The Clearness Committee: A Communal Approach to Discernment," Center for Courage and Renewal, accessed September 13, 2025, https://www

.couragerenewal.org/wp-content/uploads/2022/06/Parker-Palmer_Clearness-Committee.pdf.

Chapter 10

1. Alice M. Isen, "Success, Failure, Attention, and Reaction to Others: The Warm Glow of Success," *Journal of Personality and Social Psychology* 15 (1970): 294–301.
2. Carlos A. Estrada et al., "Positive Affect Improves Creative Problem Solving and Influences Reported Source of Practice Satisfaction in Physicians," *Motivation and Emotion* 18 (1994): 285–99.
3. Alice M. Isen and Paul F. Levin, "Effect of Feeling Good on Helping: Cookies and Kindness," *Journal of Personality and Social Psychology* 21 (1972): 384–88; Alice M. Isen and Nehemia Geva, "The Influence of Positive Affect on Acceptable Level of Risk: The Person with a Large Canoe Has a Large Worry," *Organizational Behavior and Human Decision Processes* 39 (1987): 145–54.
4. George Vaillant, *Spiritual Evolution: A Scientific Defense of Faith* (Broadway Books, 2008).
5. Robert A. Emmons, "Joy: An Introduction to This Special Issue," *The Journal of Positive Psychology* 15 (2020): 1–4.
6. Charles Mathewes, "Some Remarks on Joy," *The Journal of Positive Psychology* 15 (2020): 95–98.
7. Emmons, "Joy: An Introduction," 1.
8. Kahlil Gibran, "On Joy and Sorrow," Poets.org, accessed September 12, 2025, https://www.poets.org/poem/joy-and-sorrow.
9. Holly Harris and Michael A. Busseri, "Is There an 'End of History Illusion' for Life Satisfaction? Evidence from a Three-Wave Longitudinal Study," *Journal of Research in Personality* 83 (2019): 103869; Timothy D. Wilson and Daniel T. Gilbert, "Affective Forecasting," *Advances in Experimental Social Psychology* 35 (2003): 346–412.

10. Jordi Quoidbach et al., "The Price of Abundance: How a Wealth of Experiences Impoverishes Savoring," *Personality and Social Psychology Bulletin* 41 (2015): 393–404.
11. Karynna Okabe-Miyamoto et al., "Is Variety the Spice of Happiness? More Variety Is Associated with Lower Efficacy of Positive Activity Interventions in a Sample of over 200,000 Happiness Seekers," *The Journal of Positive Psychology* 18 (2023): 327–38.
12. Daniel Kahneman et al., "A Survey Method for Characterizing Daily Life Experience: The Day Reconstruction Method," *Science* 306 (2004): 1776–80.
13. Matthewes, "Some Remarks on Joy," 96.
14. S. Katherine Nelson-Coffey and John K. Coffey, "Gratitude Improves Parents' Well-Being and Family Functioning," *Emotion* 24 (2023): 357–69.
15. Barbara L. Fredrickson, "Positive Emotions Broaden and Build," *Advances in Experimental Social Psychology* 47 (2013): 1–53.
16. David Soto et al., "Pleasant Music Overcomes the Loss of Awareness in Patients with Visual Neglect," *Proceedings of the National Academy of Science* 106 (2009): 6011-16.
17. Eric L. Garland et al., "Upward Spirals of Positive Emotions Counter Downward Spirals of Negativity: Insights from the Broaden-and-Build Theory and Affective Neuroscience on the Treatment of Emotion Dysfunctions and Deficits in Psychopathology," *Clinical Psychology Review* 30 (2010): 849–64.
18. Barbara L. Fredrickson and Thomas Joiner, "Reflections on Positive Emotions and Upward Spirals," *Perspectives on Psychological Science* 13 (2018): 194–99.
19. Philip A. Gable and Gesine Dreisbach, "Approach Motivation and Positive Affect," *Current Opinion in Behavioral Sciences* 39 (2021): 203–8; Abigail A. Scholer et al., "Should We Approach Approach and Avoid Avoidance? An Inquiry from Different Levels," *Psychological Inquiry* 30 (2019): 111–24.

20. Paul E. Jose et al., "Savor Now and Also Reap the Rewards Later: Amplifying Savoring Predicts Greater Uplift Frequency over Time," *The Journal of Positive Psychology* 16 (2021): 738–48.
21. Brett C. Major et al., "Well-Being Correlates of Perceived Positivity Resonance: Evidence from Trait and Episode-Level Assessments," *Personality and Social Psychology Bulletin* 44 (2018): 1631–47.
22. Kelong Lu and Ning Hao, "The Interpersonal Neural Coupling in Group Creative Ideation," *Psychological Review*, 133 (2026): 221–36.
23. Uri Hasson et al., "Brain-to-Brain Coupling: A Mechanism for Creating and Sharing a Social World," *Trends in Cognitive Sciences* 16 (2012): 114–21.
24. Iris B. Mauss et al., "Don't Hide Your Happiness! Positive Emotion Dissociation, Social Connectedness, and Psychological Functioning," *Journal of Personality and Social Psychology* 100 (2011): 738–48.
25. John M. Gottman and Nan Silver, *The Seven Principles for Making Marriage Work*, 2nd ed. (Harmony Books, 2014).
26. Geoffery L. Cohen and David K. Sherman, "The Psychology of Change: Self-Affirmation and Social Psychological Intervention," *Annual Review of Psychology* 65 (2014): 333–71.
27. Geoffrey L. Cohen and David K. Sherman. "The Psychology of Change: Self-Affirmation and Social Psychological Intervention." *Annual Review of Psychology* 65 (2014): 333–71, 337.
28. Christine Logel et al., "Affirmation Prevents Long-Term Weight Gain," *Journal of Experimental Social Psychology* 81 (2019): 70–75.
29. Sumaya Albalooshi et al., "Reinstating the Resourceful Self: When and How Self-Affirmations Improve Executive Performance of the Powerless," *Personality and Social Psychology Bulletin* 46 (2020): 189–203; Brandon J. Schmeichel and Kathleen Vohs, "Self-Affirmation and Self-Control: Affirming Core Values Counteracts Ego Depletion," *Journal of Personality and Social Psychology* 96 (2009): 770–82.

Chapter 11

1. Ronald Dworkin, *Religion Without God* (Harvard University Press, 2013).
2. Charles Taylor, *Sources of the Self: The Making of Modern Identity* (Harvard University Press, 1996).
3. Václav Havel, "The Kind of Hope I Often Think About," *Disturbing the Peace: A Conversation with Karel Hvizdala*, trans. Paul Wilson (Vintage Books, 1990), 181.
4. Jane Goodall and Douglas Abrams, *The Book of Hope* (Celadon Books, 2021), 16.
5. Charlayne Hunter-Gault, "Remembering Desmond Tutu's Hope," *The New York Times*, December 27, 2021, accessed December 18, 2025, https://www.newyorker.com/news/postscript/remembering-desmond-tutus-hope.
6. John Lewis and Michael D'Orso, *Walking with the Wind: A Memoir of the Movement* (Simon & Schuster, 1998), 13.
7. Stephen G. Post, ed., *Altruism and Health: Perspectives from Empirical Research* (Oxford University Press, 2007); Sarah D. Pressman et al., "It's Good to Do Good and Receive Good: The Impact of a 'Pay It Forward' Style Kindness Intervention on Giver and Receiver Well-Being," *The Journal of Positive Psychology* 10 (2014): 293–302.

Index of Wise Practices

Tranquil Practices

Receptive Practices

Persevering Practices

Index of Wise Practices

Index

Please refer to Index of Wise Practices for practice classification by type.

Index

Index

About the Author

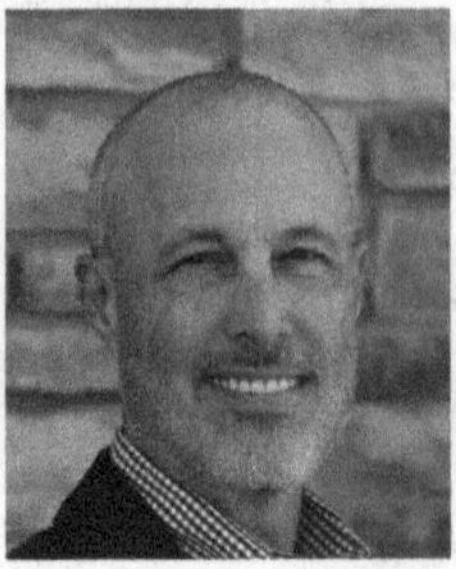

Jack Foster

Matt Bloom is a writer, speaker, entrepreneur, and emeritus professor of management at the University of Notre Dame. For over two decades, he studied the wellbeing of people in the helping and healing professions, including international aid workers, physicians, educators, and clergy. At Notre Dame, Matt taught classes on innovation to MBAs and executives. He completed his MA at the University of Kansas and his PhD at Cornell University. Some of Matt's favorite wellbeing practices are hiking, scuba diving, reading poetry, and baking bread. He lives with his wife, Kim, in Colorado.